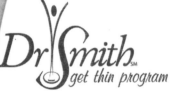

CALORIE COUNTER

The Dr. Smith Calorie Counter

Published by CreativeCommunication Publications

Distributed through *www.DrSmithProgram.com*

Copyright © 2003 by Dr. Walter Smith, DO

All rights reserved.

No part of this book may be reproduced in any form, stored in a retrieval system or translated in any form by any means— electronic, mechanical, photocopy, recording or otherwise—without prior written permission of the author, except as provided by United States of America copyright law.

DISCLAIMER

The information in this book is not intended to provide medical advice or to take the place of medical advice and treatment from your personal physician. Readers are advised to consult their own doctors or other qualified health professionals regarding the treatment of their medical problems.

2 The calorie information in this reference book is believed to be accurate as of the printing date, gathered from sources deemed to be reliable. The publisher and distributor of *The Dr. Smith Calorie Counter* are not liable for errors or omissions. Readers are encouraged to verify the caloric content of foods with food processors and vendors.

Neither the publisher nor the author takes any responsibility for any possible consequences from any treatment, action or application of medicine, supplement, herb or preparation to any person reading or following the information in this book or the Dr. Smith Get Thin Program™. If readers are taking prescription medications, they should consult with their physicians and not take themselves off of medications to start supplementation without the proper supervision of a physician.

ISBN: 0-9709307-5-5

First Edition   December, 2003

INTRODUCTION

You should be pleased with yourself — you are making a good start toward losing weight! To lose successfully and consistently, you need to learn the simple steps to counting your calories (and a couple of other things, as detailed in my book *Get Thin Now!*, based on Dr. Smith's Get Thin Program).

This *Calorie Counter* contains five parts:

- **Introduction** – which you are reading now
- **Table of Measures, Abbreviations & Types of Cooking**
- **Regular Foods** — their calorie counts
- **Eating Out** — calorie counts from restaurants and fast food chains
- **Lower Calorie Eating Out** — lower-calorie selections from restaurants and fast food chains.

The **Table of Measures, Abbreviations, and Types of Cooking** has information you might need from time to time around the kitchen or around your home place (cups, fluid ounces, gallons, tablespoons, and so on). In this section, you will find help in converting common measurements into other common measurements. It also has descriptions of the various ways to prepare foods (braise, pan fry, sautee, etc.). This might introduce you to lower calorie ways to prepare your foods.

The **Regular Foods** section contains individual food items, such as peas, chili, chicken, breads, etc., their sizes, and their calorie counts. You will notice that some foods in this section are listed with a calorie count of "basically zero." This means that by the time you chew this food you have burned about all the calories in it, so you can have all you want of these foods.

The **Eating Out** section is a listing of foods in restaurants and fast food chains with their calorie counts. When you eat out you can quickly find the calorie count of the foods you order.

The **Lower-Calorie Eating Out** section is a list of lower calorie choices at restaurants and fast food chains. If you eat out but want to quickly select the lower calorie offerings, using this section is the easy way to do that. This way you're not tempted by higher calorie foods. You can quickly look at this section, order from it, and feel great because you haven't wrecked your calories for the day. It's a wonderful lower-calorie reference for eating out.

This *Calorie Counter* will be your daily guide to get you through the world of calories. Carry this book with you — if you don't have it near you then you can't use it as a reference for your calorie counts. Keep it in your briefcase, purse, kitchen, or car. Many patients two copies, so they can have one handy wherever they might need it.

TABLE OF MEASURES & ABBREVIATIONS

qt	=	quart
c	=	cup
g	=	gram (metric system, dry weight)
ml	=	milliliter (metric system, liquid volume)
fl oz	=	fluid ounce (measures liquid volume)
oz	=	ounce (measures dry weight)
tsp	=	teaspoon
Tblsp	=	Tablespoon
gal	=	gallon
1 Tblsp	=	3 tsp
1 cup	=	8 fl oz = 16 Tblsp = 48 tsp
1/2 cup	=	4 fl oz = 8 Tblsp = 24 tsp
1/4 cup	=	2 fl oz = 4 Tblsp = 12 tsp
1 fl oz	=	2 Tblsp = 6 tsp
2 cups	=	1 pint
4 cups	=	2 pints = 1 qt
8 cups	=	4 pints = 2 qts = 1/2 gal
16 cups	=	8 pints = 4 qts = 1 gal

1 glass however, is an unknown amount!

METRIC VALUES RELATED TO AMERICAN VALUES

1/2 oz	=	14 g		
1 oz	=	28 g		
2 oz	=	57 g		
1 fl oz	=	30 ml		
1 cup	=	240 ml	=	8 fl oz
1 liter	=	33 fl oz		

Method	Description	Time	Calories
Barbequing	Cooking over open flames or hot coals where juices drip onto a hot surface to vaporize and give the traditional barbeque flavor. Wood chips can be added (usually hickory or mes-quite) to smoke and add more flavor to the food.	Short	Low
Smoking	Similar to barbequing, but the heat level is much less and the flames or coals are not anywhere close to the meat. Usually has some-thing added for flavor (liquid to evapo-rate or wood chips to give off smoke).	Long	Low
Baking	Generally done in an oven using dry continuous heat set at any range of temperature. Often the juices are captured and returned to the food in some way, either while cooking or at the table. Sometimes pastry or bread is around the food to provide something extra.	Medium to long	Medium
Broiling	Generally done in an oven using continuous very high heat. Often the juices are captured and returned to the food in some way, either while cooking or at the table.	Medium	Medium

Method	Description	Time	Calories
Braising	Browning the outside of the meat (searing) over a very high heat in a little oil, then going to a low heat in a covered pan to finish cooking.	Short	Medium
Sauteeing	Cooking over high heat in a little oil.	Short	Medium
Pan Frying	Cooking using medium heat in an amount of oil to cover the bottom of the pan about 1/4 inch or less.	Short	High
Deep Frying	Generally done in a deep solid pan, kettle, or boiler. Food is usually rolled in a batter before cooking. Requires a generous amount of oil to more than cover all the food that is placed in the pan. Requires accurate temperature control of the oil in order to properly cook the food without burning the outside coating.	Short	High

EXTRA BONUS DISCUSSION ABOUT MAKING A "PERCENT SOLUTION"

Have you ever had to make up a mixture where the instructions read something like, "Make a 2% solution"? I have, and it can be annoying and difficult. This bonus section might be of help to you in this situation.

The % number means how many units of concentrate you use for every 100 units of water. A unit can be any measure: gallons, cups, fluid ounces, and so on.

Let's use this example: "For spraying weeds, use a 1% solution." What this means is that for every 100 gallons of water, use 1 gallon of concentrate. Or for 100 cups of water, use 1 cup of concentrate. Or for every 1 gallon of water, use 1/100th of a gallon of concentrate. Whatever the amount of water, use 1/100th that amount of concentrate.

Sometimes you have to think a little bit — what amount of final mixture do you want? 100 gallons is a lot. 100 cups is also a lot (look back at the Table of Measures. 1 gallon is 16 cups, right? So 100 cups divided by 16 gives you about 6 gallons of mixture). If you needed a 1% solution in a final volume of 6 gallons, you would use 100 cups (6 gallons) of water and 1 cup of concentrate.

Maybe your sprayer only holds 2 gallons. How would you make a 1% solution? Well, cups might be a good way to start. 1 gallon = 16 cups, so 2 gallons = 32 cups. 32 cups of water in your final mixture will need 1/100th of that amount of concentrate. 32 cups divided by 100 = 0.32 cups (about 1/3 of a cup). If you wanted 2 gallons of mixture, use 2 gallons of water and 1/3rd cup of concentrate.

Now suppose the directions said to make a 3% solution. How to solve it? First, do all your calculations for making a 1% solution to find the amount of concentrate you would need for a 1% solution. Simply multiply that amount by 3 and you have the amount of concentrate needed for a 3% solution.

Let's pretend you need only 1 gallon of a 4.5% solution. Don't get nervous, just follow the examples I have already given you.

You know that your final amount is 1 gallon. You know you need a 4.5% solution. First you need to find the answer for a 1% solution. Hmmm, a gallon is a small amount, so let's do the calculations in something smaller than cups. How about fluid ounces (especially since most measuring cups are also marked in fluid ounces)?

Looking at the Table of Measures, you see that 1 gallon is 16 cups, and that 1 cup is 8 fluid ounces. That makes 16 times 8 = 128 fluid ounces in a gallon. A 1% solution would need 1.28 fluid ounces. Multiply this by 4.5 for your needed solution and you see that 5.76 (a little bit less than 6) fluid ounces will give your 4.5% solution.

There you have it — a 4.5% solution needs 1 gallon of water and 6 fluid ounces of concentrate.

I hope these examples help you.

Dr. Walter Smith, DO

10

Alphabetical List of Foods	Calories
Abalone – fried	4 oz = 215
Almonds – fresh	1/4 c sliced = 135
Almonds – dry roasted	1/4 c = 205
Anchovy – canned In oil	10 = 100
Apple Juice – canned or bottled, unsweetened	1 c = 115
Apple Juice – frozen concentrate, unsweetened made with water	1 c = 110
Apple Juice – unsweetened	1 c = 115
Apple Sauce – canned, sweetened	1 c = 195
Apple Sauce – canned, sweetened	1/2 c = 95
Apple Sauce – canned, unsweetened	1 c = 105
Apple Sauce – canned, unsweetened	1/2 c = 50
Apples – fresh	1 = 75
Apricot Nectar – canned	1 c = 140
Apricots – canned w/heavy syrup	1/2 c = 105
Apricots – canned w/light Syrup	1/2 c = 80
Apricots – fresh	1/2 c = 35
Archway Cookies – Ginger Snaps	1 = 25
Archway Cookies – Home Style, All Except Ginger And Lemon Snaps	1 = 110 average
Archway Cookies – Iced Ginger Snaps	1 = 35
Archway Cookies – Lemon Snaps	1 = 30
Armour Corned Beef Hash – canned	1 serving = 500
Artichoke Hearts – boiled	1/2 c = 40
Arugula – fresh (basically zero)	0
Asparagus – boiled (basically zero)	0
Avocados – fresh	1/2 c cubes = 120
Bacon – Canadian-style, grilled	2 slices = 85
Bacon – cooked	3 slices = 110
Bagels, plain, onion, poppy, sesame, egg cinnamon, raisin, oat	1 large = 315
	1 small = 190
Bamboo Shoots – boiled (basically zero)	0
Bananas – fresh, uncooked	1 = 80
Banquet Chicken & Potatoes Pie – Frozen	1 serving = 380
Banquet brand Meals:	
Banquet Salisbury Steak Meal, w/gravy, mashed potatoes, corn	1 serving = 400
Banquet Sliced Beef Meal w/gravy mashed potatoes, peas	1 serving = 270
Banquet Turkey & Gravy w/dressing, mashed potatoes, corn	1 serving = 280
Banquet Veal Parmigiana w/mashed potatoes, peas	1 serving = 360
Banquet, Original Fried Chicken Meal w/mashed potatoes, corn	1 serving = 470
Barley – cooked	1 c = 195

BEANS – BREADS

Beans, Baked – canned, without pork	1 c = 235
Beans, Baked – canned, w/pork	1 c = 270
Beans, Baked– home prepared	1 c = 380
Beans – snap, green, cooked, fresh frozen or canned	1 c = 40
Beans – snap, yellow, canned	1 c = 25
Beef Potatoes Pie – frozen entree	1 serving = 450
Beef Stew – canned	1 serving = 220
Beef (cooked)	
Beef, Bottom Round – cooked	4 oz = 240
Beef, Bottom Sirloin, Tri-tip – cooked	4 oz = 235
Beef, Brisket – cooked	4 oz = 245
Beef, Chuck Roast – cooked	4 oz = 345
Beef, Corned Beef Brisket – cooked	4 oz = 285
Beef, Eye of Round – cooked	4 oz = 195
Beef, Ground Hamburger Patties	4 oz = 320
Beef, Hamburger Patties – precooked	1 serving = 160
Beef, Pastrami	1 slice = 100
Beef, Porterhouse Steak – cooked	10 oz steak = 780
Beef, Ribs – cooked	4 oz meat = 345
Beef, T-bone Steak – cooked	10 oz steak = 780
Beef, Tenderloin – cooked	1 steak = 220
Beef, Tongue – cooked,	4 oz = 320
Beef, Top Round – cooked	4 oz = 240
Beef, Top Sirloin – cooked	4 oz = 245
Beets – cooked or canned	1 c = 40
Beets, Pickled – canned	1 c slices = 150
Best Foods Thomas' English Muffins – plain	1 = 130
Betty Crocker Hamburger Helper, Cheeseburger	1 serving = 180
Biscuit w/egg & sausage	1 = 580
Biscuit w/egg & steak	1 = 410
Biscuits – home-baked	1 = 130
Biscuits – homemade	1 = 360
Blackberries – canned, heavy syrup	1/2 c = 120
Blackberries – fresh	1/2 c = 40
Blueberries – canned, heavy syrup	1/2 c = 115
Blueberries – frozen, sweetened	1/2 c = 95
Blueberries – frozen, unsweetened	1/2 c = 40
Blueberries – fresh	1/2 c = 40
Bologna	1 oz = 95
	1 slice = 70
Bologna Lite	1 oz = 60
Boysenberries – canned, heavy syrup	1/2 c = 115
Boysenberries – frozen, unsweetened	1/2 c = 35
Bratwurst	1 = 255, 1 oz = 85
Brazil nuts, Dried, Shelled	1/4 c = 230
Breads	
Bread Sticks, Plain	1 stick = 20
Banana, Home Made	4 oz slice = 370
Cornbread, Home Cooked	4 oz piece = 330
Egg	1 thin slice = 115

French	1 slice = 175
Italian	1 slice = 80
Mixed-Grain	1 slice = 80
Pita	1 pita = 170
Pumpernickel	1 slice = 80
Raisin	1 slice = 90
Raisin – enriched	1 slice = 85
Rye	1 slice = 80
Sourdough	1 slice = 175
Wheat	1 slice = 65
White	1 slice = 85
Breakfast Burrito, Ham & Cheese Flavor	1 serving = 210
Broccoli, fresh or cooked	1 c = 25, 1 stalk = 60
Brownies – prebaked	1 = 225
Brownies – home-baked from a mix	1 = 270
Brownies – homemade	1 = 110
Brussels Sprouts – fresh or cooked	1 c = 60
Budget Gourmet brand meals	
Budget Gourmet Light & Healthy Salisbury Steak	
w/potatoes & vegetables	1 serving = 260
Budget Gourmet Light & Healthy Teryaki Chicken	
w/vegetables	1 serving = 317
Budget Gourmet Light Chicken w/vegetables,	
potatoes, wine sauce	1 serving = 180
Butter	1/2 cup = 405
	1 tsp = 35
	1 Tblsp = 100
Cabbage – cooked	1/2 c = 155
Cakes	
Angelfood	1 slice = 75
Boston Cream Pie	1 piece = 230
Chocolate w/chocolate frosting	
– prebaked	1 piece = 235
Fruitcake – prebaked	1 piece = 140
Gingerbread – homemade	1 piece = 265
Pineapple Upside-Down – homemade	1 piece = 365
Pound – prebaked	1 piece = 110
Shortcake – biscuit-type, homemade	1 biscuit = 100
Snack Cakes – creme-filled, sponge	1 piece = 155
Sponge – prebaked	1 piece = 110
White – without frosting, homemade	1 piece = 265
White – w/coconut frosting, homemade	1 piece = 400
Yellow – without frosting, homemade	1 piece = 245
Yellow – with chocolate or vanilla frosting	
— prebaked	1 piece = 240
Candies	
M&M's Peanut Chocolate Candy	1/2 c = 440
M&M's Plain Chocolate Candy	1/2 c = 510
3 Musketeers Bar	1 = 210
5th Avenue Bar	1 regular = 270

CANDIES – CEREALS

Almond Joy Bites	10 = 120
Almond Joy Bar	1 regular package = 235
Butterscotch	5 = 100
Caramels	5 = 200
Chocolate-covered raisins	1/2 c = 350
Fudge – homemade	1 piece = 70
Heath Bites	10 = 140
Jellybeans	10 regular = 105, 10 small = 40
Kit Kat Bar	1 med size = 290
Kit Kat Bites	10 = 135
Mars Almond Bar	1 = 235
Mars Milky Way Bar	1 regular = 270
Milk Chocolate w/almonds	1 bar = 220
Mounds Bar	1 regular = 240
Mr. Goodbar	1 regular = 265
Nestle 100 Grand Bar	1 = 200
Nestle Baby Ruth Bar	1 regular = 165
Nestle Butterfinger	1 regular = 215
Nestle Chunky Bar	1 = 190
Nestle Crunch Bar	1 = 210
Nestle Goobers	10 = 250
Nestle Oh Henry! Bar	1 = 245
Reese Bites	10 = 125
Reese's Peanut Butter Cups	1 small = 35, 5 = 175
Reese's Pieces	10 = 40
Rolo Caramels	2 rolls (3 pieces each) = 170
Skor Toffee Bar	1 bar = 1210
Snickers Bar	1 = 275
Sugar-coated Almonds	10 = 160
Twix Caramel	1 package = 285
Twix Peanut Butter	1 package = 305
Willy Wonka's Everlasting Gobstoppers	1 = 10
York Peppermint Pattie	1 = 165
Carrot Juice, Canned	1 c = 95
Carrots, fresh or cooked (basically zero)	0
Castleberry Premium Beef Stew, Canned	1 serving = 330
Catsup (Ketchup) (basically zero)	0
Cauliflower, fresh or cooked (basically zero)	0
Caviar	1 Tblsp = 40
Celery, fresh or cooked (basically zero)	0
Celeste Deluxe Pizza w/sausage & peppers – frozen	1 serving = 386
Cereals (Generic Brands)	
Cream of Wheat (stove-cooked)	1 c = 135
Cream of Wheat, Instant	1 c = 155
Cream of Wheat, Instant, All Flavors	1 c = 155
Cream of Wheat, Mix'n Eat, All Flavors	1 c = 130
Cream of Wheat, Quick	1 c = 130
Cream of Wheat, Regular or Quick	1 c = 130
Crispy Rice	1 c = 110

CEREALS

Farina	1 c = 115
Cereals (General Mills)	
General Mills Apple Cinnamon Cheerios	1 c = 155
General Mills Basic 4	1 c = 200
General Mills Berry Berry Kix	1 c = 155
General Mills Boo Berry	1 c = 120
General Mills Cheerios	1 c = 110
General Mills Cinnamon Toast Crunch	1 c = 170
General Mills Cocoa Puffs	1 c = 115
General Mills Cookie Crisp	1 c = 115
General Mills Corn Chex	1 c = 110
General Mills Count Chocula	1 c = 120
General Mills Country Corn Flakes	1 c = 110
General Mills Fiber One	1 c = 120
General Mills Frankenberry	1 c = 120
General Mills Frosted Wheaties	1 c = 150
General Mills Golden Grahams	1 c = 150
General Mills Honey Nut Cheerios	1 c = 110
General Mills Honey Nut Chex	1 c = 150
General Mills Honey Nut Clusters	1 c = 215
General Mills Kaboom	1 c = 90
General Mills Kix	1 c = 85
General Mills Lucky Charms	1 c = 115
General Mills Muliti-grain Chex	1 c = 165
General Mills Multi-grain Cheerios	1 c = 110
General Mills Oatmeal Crisp With Almonds	1 c = 220
General Mills Oatmeal Crisp With Apples	1 c = 205
General Mills Oatmeal Raisin Crisp	1 c = 205
General Mills Raisin Nut Bran	1 c = 210
General Mills Reese's Puffs	1 c = 170
General Mills Rice Chex	1 c = 95
General Mills Total Corn Flakes	1 c = 85
General Mills Total Raisin Bran	1 c = 170
General Mills Trix	1 c = 115
General Mills Wheat Chex	1 c = 105
General Mills Wheaties	1 c = 110
General Mills Wheaties Raisin Bran	1 c = 185
General Mills Whole Grain Total	1 c = 130
Cereals (Heartland brand)	
Heartland Natural Cereal – plain	1 c = 500
Heartland Natural Cereal – w/coconut	1 c = 465
Heartland Natural Cereal – w/raisins	1 c = 470
Cereals (Kellogg's brand)	
Kellogg's All-Bran	1 c = 100
Kellogg's All-Bran	1 c = 160
Kellogg's All-Bran Bran Buds	1 c = 150
Kellogg's Apple Cinnamon Squares Mini-Wheats	1 c = 240
Kellogg's Apple Jacks	1 c = 115
Kellogg's Cocoa Krispies	1 c = 155
Kellogg's Complete Oat Bran Flakes	1 c = 140

CEREALS

Kellogg's Complete Wheat Bran Flakes	1 c = 120
Kellogg's Corn Flakes	1 c = 100
Kellogg's Corn Pops	1 c = 120
Kellogg's Cracklin' Oat Bran	1 c = 300
Kellogg's Crispix	1 c = 110
Kellogg's Froot Loops	1 c = 120
Kellogg's Frosted Flakes	1 c = 150
Kellogg's Frosted Mini-Wheats, Bite Size	1 c = 190
Kellogg's Frosted Mini-Wheats, Original	1 c = 175
Kellogg's Frosted Rice Krispies	1 c = 150
Kellogg's Honey Crunch Corn Flakes	1 c = 155
Kellogg's Just Right Fruit & Nut	1 c = 220
Kellogg's Lo Fat Granola — no raisins	1 c = 370
Kellogg's Lo Fat Granola w/raisins	1 c = 345
Kellogg's Mueslix	1 c = 295
Kellogg's Product 19	1 c = 110
Kellogg's Raisin Bran	1 c = 190
Kellogg's Raisin Bran Crunch	1 c = 190
Kellogg's Raisin Squares Mini-Wheats	1 c = 245
Kellogg's Rice Krispies	1 c = 100
Kellogg's Rice Krispies Treats Cereal	1 c = 160
Kellogg's Smacks	1 c = 140
Kellogg's Smart Start	1 c = 182
Kellogg's Special K	1 c = 115
Kellogg's Special K Red Berries	1 c = 115
Kellogg's Strawberry Mini-Wheats	1 c = 225
Cereals (Maltex brand)	
Maltex	1 c = 180
Malt-o-Meal Berry Colossal Crunch	1 c = 160
Malt-o-Meal Colossal Crunch	1 c = 160
Malt-o-Meal Corn Bursts	1 c = 120
Malt-o-Meal Crispy Rice	1 c = 125
Malt-o-Meal Plain & Chocolate	1 c = 120
Malt-o-Meal Toasty O's	1 c = 110
Malt-o-Meal Tootie Fruities	1 c = 125
Cereal (Nature Valley brand)	
Nature Valley Lo Fat Fruit Granola	1 c = 35
Cereals (Post brand)	
Post 100% Bran	1 c = 250
Post Banana Nut Crunch	1 c = 250
Post Blueberry Morning	1 c = 170
Post Bran Flakes	1 c = 130
Post Cocoa Pebbles	1 c = 155
Post Frosted Alpha-bits	1 c = 130
Post Frosted Shredded Wheat Bite Size	1 c = 185
Post Fruit & Fibre w/dates, raisins & walnuts	1 c = 210
Post Fruity Pebbles	1 c = 145
Post Golden Crisp	1 c = 140
Post Grape-Nuts (Original)	1 c = 415
Post Grape-Nuts Flakes	1 c = 140

Post Great Grains Crunchy Pecan	1 c = 325
Post Great Grains Raisin, Date & Pecan	1 c = 305
Post Honey Bunches of Oats Honey Roasted	1 c = 155
Post Honey Bunches of Oats w/almonds	1 c = 170
Post Honeycomb	1 c = 85
Post Marshmallow Alpha-Bits	1 c = 115
Post Oreo O's	1 c = 150
Post Raisin Bran	1 c = 185
Post The Origin Shredded Wheat Spoon Size	1 c = 165
Post The Original Shredded Wheat	2 biscuits = 155
Post The Original Shredded Wheat 'n Bran	1 c = 160
Post Toasties Corn Flakes	1 c = 100
Post Waffle Crisp	1 c = 130
Cereals (Quaker brand)	
Quaker 100% Natural Cereal with Oats, Honey & Raisins	1 c = 450
Quaker 100% Natural Granola Oats & Honey	1 c = 465
Quaker Apple Zaps	1 c = 155
Quaker Cap'n Crunch	1 c = 145
Quaker Cap'n Crunch With Crunchberries	1 c = 140
Quaker Cap'n Crunch's Peanut Butter Crunch	1 c = 150
Quaker Cinnamon Oatmeal Squares	1 c = 225
Quaker Cocoa Blasts	1 c = 130
Quaker Cranberry Macadamia Nut	1 c = 245
Quaker Crunchy Bran	1 c = 120
Quaker Honey Graham Oh!s	1 c = 150
Quaker Honey Nut Heaven	1 c = 190
Quaker King Vitaman	1 c = 80
Quaker Lo-Fat 100% Natural Granola w/raisins	1 c = 390
Quaker Multigrain Oatmeal, Dry	1 c = 265
Quaker Oat Cinnamon Life	1 c = 160
Quaker Oat Life, Plain	1 c = 160
Quaker Oatmeal Squares	1 c = 210
Quaker Puffed Rice	1 c = 55
Quaker Puffed Wheat	1 c = 45
Quaker Sweet Puffs	1 c = 135
Cereal, Sun Country Granola w/almonds	1 c = 530
Cereal, Waffelos	1 c = 120
Cereal, Puffed Rice	1 c = 55
Cereal, Wheat Germ, Toasted, Plain	1 c = 430
Cereal, Puffed Wheat	1 c = 45
Cereal, Wheat, Shredded, Plain	1 rectangular biscuit = 80
Cereal, Wheatena	1 c = 135
Cheese Spread, Pasteurized Process	1/2 c diced = 205
	1/2 c solid = 355
Cheeses	
Cheese, Blue	1 oz = 100
	1 cubic inch = 60
Cheese, Brie	1/2 c melted = 400
	shredded = 210

Cheese, Camembert	1/2 c = 370
	1 oz = 85
Cheese, Cheddar	1/2 c: diced = 265
	melted = 490
Cheese, Cottage, non-fat & low-fat	1/2 c = 80
	4 oz = 100
Cheese, Cottage, Regular	1/2 c = 110
	4 oz = 115
Cheese, Cream	1 tsp = 50
	1/2 c = 405
Cheese, Feta	1 oz = 75
	1/2 c crumbled = 200
Cheese, Goat	1 oz = 100
Cheese, Gouda	1 oz = 100
	1 cubic inch = 60
Cheese, Mozzarella, Whole Milk	1 oz = 80
	1/2 c shredded = 160
Cheese, Parmesian	1/2 c grated = 230
	shredded = 170
	1 Tblsp = 25
Cheese, Pasteurized Process, American	1/2 c diced = 265
	melted = 460
Cheese, Pasteurized Process, Pimento	1/2 c diced = 265
	melted = 460
Cheese, Pasteurized Process, Swiss	1/2 c diced = 235
	shredded = 190
Cheese, Provolone	1 oz = 100
	1/2 c = 230
Cheese, Ricotta, Whole Milk	1 oz = 50
	1/2 cp = 215
Cheese, Roquefort	1 oz = 105
Cheese, Swiss	1/2 c diced = 250
	melted = 460
Cheesecakes	
Cheesecake – prebaked	1 piece = 255
Cheesecake – no-bake type, homemade	1 piece = 270
Chef Boyardee products	
Chef Boyardee Beef Ravioli, canned	1 serving = 230
Chef Boyardee Beefaroni, canned	1 serving = 185
Chef Boyardee Mini Ravioli, canned	1 serving = 240
Chef Boyardee Spaghetti & Meatballs – canned	1 serving = 250
Chef Boyardee Teen Ninja Turtle Pasta & Meatballs – canned	1 serving = 225
Cherries, Sweet, fresh	1/2 c = 40
Chewing Gum	1 stick = 10
	10 chicklets = 55
Chicken & Potatoes Pie, Frozen Entrée	1 serving = 485
Chicken Breast Roll	1 oz = 35

Chicken, Fried, Drumstick	meat and skin = 195
	meat only = 80
Chicken, Fried, Thigh	meat and skin = 240
	meat only = 115
Chicken, Fried, Whole Breast	meat and skin = 730
	meat only = 320
Chicken, Fried, Wing	meat and skin = 160
	meat only = 40
Chicken Gizzard – simmered (not fried)	1 c = 200
Chicken Liver – simmered (not fried)	1 c = 200
Chicken, Roasted, Drumstick	meat and skin = 115
	meat only = 50
Chicken, Roasted, Thigh	meat and skin = 145
	meat only = 70
Chicken, Roasted, Whole Breast	meat and skin = 440
	meat only = 190
Chicken, Roasted, Wing	meat and skin = 95
	meat only = 25
Chili Con Carne w/beans – canned	1 serving = 255
Chili w/beans – canned	1 c = 285
Chips, Corn	10 = 130
Chocolate Syrup	1 Tblsp = 160
Chorizo	1 = 275
Chowder, Clam, Manhattan (canned)	1 c mixed w/water = 80
Chowder, Clam, New England (canned)	1 c mixed w/milk = 95
Chowder, Clam, New England (canned)	1 c mixed w/water = 95
Chowder, Clam – Progresso Brand New English	1 c = 115
Chun King Sweet & Sour Vegetables Fruit & Sauce	
w/chicken (canned)	1 serving = 165
Cinnamon Swirl French Toast w/Sausage	1 serving = 415
Clams, Breaded & Fried	4 oz = 230
Clams, Cooked Not Fried	4 oz = 170
Cocoa Mix, Nestle, Carnation	1 serving = 110
Coconut Meat, Flakes – dried, sweetened	1 oz =125
Coconut Meat – fresh	1/4 c = 70
Coconut Milk – canned	1 c = 445
Coffeecakes	
Cheese Coffeecake	1 piece = 260
Cinnamon Coffeecake w/crumb topping	
– premade	1 piece = 240
Collards, Cooked	1 c = 50
Cookies (Generic brands)	
Butter – premade	1 = 25
Chocolate Chip – prebaked	1 = 50
Chocolate Chip – home-baked	1 = 80
Chocolate Chip – refrigerated dough, home-baked	1 = 60
Chocolate Chip – soft-type,prebaked	1 = 70
Chocolate Sandwich w/creme filling	1 = 45
Coconut Macaroons – home-baked	1 = 95
Fig Bars	1 bar = 150

Fortune	1 = 30
Fudge – cake-type	1 = 75
Gingersnaps	1 = 30
Graham Crackers – chocolate-coated	1 square = 70
Graham Crackers – plain, cinnamon or honey	1 square = 15
Ladyfingers	1 = 45
Oatmeal – prebaked	1 = 115
Oatmeal – prebaked, fat-free	1 = 90
Oatmeal – home-baked	1 = 70
Oatmeal – refrigerated dough, home-baked	1 = 55
Oatmeal – w/raisins, home-baked	1 = 65
Peanut Butter – prebaked	1 = 70
Peanut Butter – home-baked	1 = 95
Peanut Butter – refrigerated dough, home-baked	1 = 60
Shortbread – pecan, pre-baked	1 = 75
Sugar Wafers w/creme filling	1 = 45
Sugar – prebaked	1 = 70
Sugar – homemade	1 = 65
Sugar – refrigerated dough, home-baked	1 = 110
Vanilla Wafers	1 = 30
Corn, Sweet, Yellow or White – Boiled	1 ear = 85
	1 c kernels = 175
Corned Beef Loaf	1 slice = 45
Cornish Game Hen – meat w/skin – roasted	1 = 770
Cornish Game Hen – meat only – roasted	1 = 294
Cornnuts	1/2c = 195
Couscous – cooked	1 c = 175
Crab	
Crab Cakes – cooked	1 = 95
Crab, Alaska King – cooked	1 leg = 130
Crab, Blue – cooked or canned	1 c = 130
Crab, Dungeness – cooked (not fried)	4 oz = 125
Crackers, Melba Toast, Plain, Rye, Wheat or Pumpernickel	1 toast = 20
Crackers, saltines	1 = 10
Crackers, saltines – fat-free	1 = 20
Crackers – whole-wheat	1 = 20
Cranberry Sauce – canned, sweetened	2 Tblsp = 50
Crayfish – cooked	4 oz = 95
Cream Puff – homemade	1 = 335
Cream and Creamers	
Cream Substitute – liquid	1 Tblsp = 20
	1/2 c = 165
Cream, Half-and-Half®	1 Tblsp = 20
Cream – Heavy Whipping	1/2 c non-whipped liquid = 410
	whipped = 205
Cream – Light Whipping	1/2 c non-whipped liquid = 350
	whipped = 175
Cream, Sour	1/2 c = 245
	1 Tblsp = 25

CREAM – DRINKS

Cream, Whipped (pressurized can)	1/2 c = 75
	1 Tblsp = 8
Croissants	1 = 115
Croutons, Plain	1/4 c = 30
Cucumber, fresh (basically zero)	0
Dandelion Greens – cooked (basically zero)	0
Danish Pastry, Dry, Cinnamon, Cheese, Fruit or Nut	1 = 280
Dates, Domestic	1/2 c = 245
Doughnuts – various types	
Cake-type – chocolate-coated	1 = 250
Cake-type – chocolate, sugared or glazed	1 = 250
Cake-type – plain	1 = 220
Cake-type – sugared or glazed	1 = 190
French Cruller – Glazed	1 = 170
Glazed	1 = 250
Glazed – w/creme filling	1 = 305
Glazed – w/jelly filling	1 = 290
Drink, Alcoholic – various types	
Beer, Light	1 can = 100
Beer, Regular	1 can = 145
Daiquiri – canned	1 c = 305
Daiquiri – homemade	1 c = 450
Gin, Rum, Vodka, Whiskey	1 jigger = 105
Liqueur, Coffee	1 jigger = 175
Liqueur, Coffee w/cream	1 jigger = 155
Pina Colada – canned	1 c = 615
Pina Colada – homemade	1 c = 450
Tequila Sunrise – canned	1 c = 270
Whiskey Sour	1 c = 150
Wine – all	1/2 c = 85
Wine – dessert, sweet	1/2 c = 180
Drink, Carbonated – various types	
Club Soda (basically zero)	0
Cola	1 can = 200
Cream Soda	1 can = 250
Ginger Ale	1 can = 165
Grape Soda	1 can = 160
Lemon-Lime Soda	1 can = 195
Orange Soda	1 can = 240
"Pepper" type	1 can = 200
Root Beer	1 can = 200
Drink, Miscellaneous	
Clam & Tomato Juice – canned	1 c = 110
Cocoa Mix – sugar-free	1 serving = 55
Coffee – without sugar or cream (basically zero)	0
Cranberry Juice Cocktail	1 c = 145
Cranberry Juice Cocktail – low-calorie	1 c = 45
Cranberry-Apple Juice	1 c = 165
Cranberry-Apricot Juice	1 c = 155
Cranberry-Grape Juice	1 c = 135

DRINKS – FAST FOODS

Grape Drink – canned (not Grape Juice)	1 c = 115
Lemonade, Pink – frozen concentrate mix	
made w/water	1 c = 100
Lemonade – powder mix, made w/water	1 c = 105
Limeade – frozen concentrate mix, made w/water	1 c = 100
Milkshake – fast food chocolate	2 c = 420
Milkshake – fast food strawberry	2 c = 510
Milkshake – fast food vanilla	2 c = 370
Orange Drink – canned	1 c = 125
Pineapple & Orange Juice	1 c = 125
Strawberry-flavor – powder mix, made w/milk	1 c = 235
Tea – brewed or instant, without sugar (basically zero)	0
Tea – brewed or instant, sweetened w/sugar	1 c = 85
Duck, meat w/skin, roasted	1 c chopped = 470
	1/4 duck = 625
Duck, meat only, roasted	1 c chopped = 280
	1/4 duck = 375
Eclairs, custard-filled w/chocolate glaze – homemade	1 = 295
Eel – cooked, not fried	4 oz fillet = 270
Eggs products	
Egg substitute – liquid	1/2 c = 100
Egg – whole, fried	1 large = 100
Egg – whole, hard-boiled	1 large = 85
Egg – whole, poached	1 large = 75
Egg – whole, scrambled	1 large = 85
Eggnog	1 c = 345
Eggplant – cooked, boiled	1 c = 305
English Muffins – all types	1 = 140
Falafel	1/4 c = 105
Fast Food Items	
Biscuit w/egg	1 = 375
Biscuit w/egg & bacon	1 = 460
Biscuit w/egg & ham	1 = 440
Biscuit w/egg, cheese & bacon	1 = 475
Biscuit w/ham	1 = 385
Biscuit w/sausage	1 = 485
Brownie	1 = 245
Burrito w/beans	1 = 255
Burrito w/beans & cheese	1 = 190
Burrito w/beans & chili peppers	1 = 205
Burrito w/beans & meat	1 = 255
Burrito w/beans, cheese & beef	1 = 165
Burrito w/beans, cheese & chili peppers	1 = 330
Burrito w/beef	1 = 260
Burrito w/beef & chili peppers	1 = 215
Burrito w/beef, cheese & chili peppers	1 = 315
Cheeseburger – large	1 = 610
Cheeseburger – large, double-meat	1 = 705
Cheeseburger – regular size	1 = 320
Cheeseburger – regular size, double-meat	1 = 455

FAST FOODS

Chicken – boneless breast sandwich	1 = 515
Chicken – breaded & fried, dark meat	2 pieces = 430
Chicken – breaded & fried, light Meat	2 pieces = 495
Chicken, Nuggets, Breaded & Fried	6 = 320
Chili Con Carne	1 c = 256
Chimichanga w/beef	1 = 425
Chimichanga w/beef & cheese	1 = 445
Chimichanga w/beef & chili peppers	1 = 425
Chimichanga w/beef, cheese & chili peppers	1 = 365
Clams – breaded & fried	1 c = 600
Coleslaw	1/2 c = 100
Cookies – chocolate chip	1 box = 235
Corn on the Cob, w/butter	1 = 155
Crab Cake	1 = 160
Croissant w/egg & cheese	1 = 370
Croissant w/egg, cheese & bacon	1 = 415
Croissant w/egg, cheese & ham	1 = 475
Croissant w/egg, cheese & sausage	1 = 525
Danish – pasteurized, cheese or cinnamon	1 = 355
Danish – pasteurized, fruit	1 = 335
Egg – scrambled	1 = 100
Enchilada w/cheese	1 = 320
Enchilada w/cheese & beef	1 = 325
Enchirito w/cheese, beef & beans	1 = 345
English Muffin w/butter	1 = 190
English Muffin w/cheese & sausage	1 = 395
English Muffin w/egg, cheese & Canadian bacon	1 = 290
English Muffin w/egg, cheese & sausage	1 = 485
Fish Fillet – battered or breaded, fried	1 = 210
Fish Sandwich w/tartar sauce	1 = 430
French Fries	1 large = 580
French Toast Sticks	5 = 515
Frijoles w/cheese	1 = 225
Ham & Cheese sandwich	1 = 350
Ham, egg & cheese sandwich	1 = 345
Hamburger – large	1 = 425
Hamburger – large, double-meat	1 = 540
Hamburger – regular size	1 = 275
Hamburger – regular size, double-meat	1 = 545
Hotdog	1 = 240
Hotdog w/chili	1 = 295
Hush Puppies	1 = 50
Ice Milk – vanilla, soft-serve w/cone	1 = 165
Nachos w/cheese	1 serving = 345
Nachos w/cheese, beans, ground beef & peppers	1 serving = 570
Nachos w/cinnamon & sugar	1 serving = 590
Onion Rings – breaded & fried	1 serving = 275
Oysters – battered or breaded, fried	6 = 370
Pancakes w/butter & syrup	1 = 260

Pizza – various styles	
Pizza w/cheese	1 slice = 140
Pizza w/cheese, meat & vegetables	1 slice = 185
Pizza w/pepperoni	1 slice = 180
Potato Salad	1/2 c = 160
Potato – baked & topped w/cheese	1 = 475
Potato – baked & topped w/cheese & bacon	1 = 451
Potato – baked & topped w/cheese & broccoli	1 = 405
Potato – baked & topped w/cheese & chili	1 = 482
Potato – baked & topped w/sour cream & chives	1 = 395
Potatoes – hashed brown	1/2 c = 150
Potatoes – mashed	1/2 c = 100
Roast Beef Sandwich	1 = 345
Roast Beef Sandwich w/cheese	1 = 475
Salads – various styles	
Salad without dressing	2 c = 45
Salad without dressing, w/cheese & egg	2 c = 135
Salad without dressing, w/pasta & seafood	2 c = 505
Salad without dressing, w/shrimp	2 c = 140
Salad without dressing, w/turkey, ham & cheese	2 c = 355
Salad without dressing, w/chicken	2 c = 140
Shrimp, Breaded & Fried	5 large = 100
Steak Sandwich	1 = 460
Submarine Sandwiches – various styes	
Submarine Sandwich w/cold cuts	1 = 455
Submarine Sandwich w/roast beef	1 = 410
Submarine Sandwich w/tuna salad	1 = 585
Various Sundaes	
Sundae, Caramel	1 = 305
Sundae, Hot Fudge	1 = 285
Sundae, Strawberry	1 = 270
Taco	1 large = 570
Taco Salad	1.5 c = 280
Taco Salad With Chili	1.5 c = 290
Tostada w/beans & cheese	1 = 225
Tostada w/beans, beef & cheese	1 = 335
Tostada w/beef & cheese	1 = 315
Figs – canned, in heavy syrup	1/2 c = 115
Figs – canned, in light syrup	1/2 c = 85
Figs – canned, in water	1/2 c = 65
Figs – fresh	1 = 40
Fish – various types	
Bass – fresh water, cooked (not fried)	4 oz fillet = 130
Catfish – breaded & fried	4 oz fillet = 260
Cod – cooked (not fried)	4 oz fillet = 120
Croaker – breaded & fried	4 oz fillet = 250
Gefilte Fish – cooked (not fried)	1 piece = 35
Grouper – cooked (not fried)	4 oz fillet = 130
Haddock – cooked (not fried)	4 oz fillet = 125
Halibut – cooked (not fried)	4 oz fillet = 160

FISH – GELATIN

Herring – cooked (not fried)	4 oz fillet = 230
Herring – kippered	1 oz = 60
Herring – pickled	1/4 c = 90
Mackerel – Atlantic Spanish or King, cooked (not fried)	4 oz fillet = 400
Mullet – cooked (not fried)	4 oz fillet = 170
Perch – ocean and fresh water cooked (not fried)	4 oz fillet = 135
Pike – Northern and Walleye cooked (not fried)	4 oz fillet = 130
Pompano – cooked (not fried)	4 oz fillet = 240
Rockfish – cooked (not fried)	4 oz fillet = 135
Roughy, Orange – cooked (not fried)	4 oz fillet = 80
Salmon – fresh or canned in water cooked (not fried)	4 oz fillet = 150
Sardine – canned in oil	1/4 c = 80
Sardine – canned in tomato sauce	1/4 c = 40
Sea Bass – cooked (not fried)	4 oz fillet = 140
Snapper – cooked (not fried)	4 oz fillet = 145
Swordfish – cooked (not fried)	4 oz fillet = 175
Trout, Rainbow – cooked (not fried)	4 oz fillet = 170
Tuna Salad	1 c = 385
Tuna – canned in oil	3 oz = 165
Tuna – canned In water	3 oz = 120
Tuna – cooked (not fried)	4 oz fillet = 210
Turbot – cooked (not fried)	4 oz fillet = 140
Whitefish – cooked (not fried)	4 oz fillet = 125
Whiting – cooked (not fried)	4 oz fillet = 130
Yellowtail – cooked (not fried)	4 oz fillet = 210
Frankfurter – beef, chicken & pork	1 = 140
Frankfurter – pork	1 - 205
Frankfurter – turkey	1 = 100
French Toast – homemade	1 slice = 150
Fruit Cocktail – canned in heavy syrup	1/2 c = 90
Fruit Cocktail – canned in juice	1/2 c = 55
Fruit Cocktail – canned in light syrup	1/2 c = 70
Game Meat – various types	
Antelope – cooked (not fried)	4 oz = 170
Beefalo – cooked (not fried)	4 oz = 415
Bison – cooked (not fried)	4 oz = 165
Boar – cooked (not fried)	4 oz = 180
Caribou – cooked (not fried)	4 oz = 190
Deer – cooked (not fried)	4 oz = 180
Elk – cooked (not fried)	4 oz = 165
Goat – cooked (not fried)	4 oz = 165
Moose – cooked (not fried)	4 oz = 150
Rabbit – cooked (not fried)	4 oz = 230
Squirrel – cooked (not fried)	4 oz = 195
Water Buffalo – cooked (not fried)	4 oz = 150
Gelatin Dessert – dry mix, home-cooked w/water	1 c = 325

GOOSE – HEALTHY CHOICE

Goose – meat & skin, roasted	1 c chopped = 425
	1/4 goose = 1250
Goose – meat only, roasted	1 c chopped = 340
	1/4 goose = 750
Granola Bars – hard or soft, plain	1 = 120
Granola Bars – hard, almond, chocolate chip, peanut butter, raisin, coated	1 = 125
Granola Bars – hard, peanut	1 = 135
Granola Bars – soft, chocolate-coated, peanut butter	1 = 185
Grape Juice – canned or bottled, unsweetened	1 c = 155
Grape Juice, from frozen concentrate sweetened made w/water	1 c = 130
Grape Leaves – canned (basically zero)	0
Grapefruit Juice – canned, sweetened	1 c = 115
Grapefruit Juice – canned, unsweetened	1 c = 95
Grapefruit – fresh	1/2 = 55
Grapes – red or green or purple, Fresh	1 c = 115
Gravy - various types	
Au Jus – canned	1 c = 40
	2 Tblsp = 5
Beef – canned	1 c = 125
	2 Tblsp = 15
Chicken – canned	1 c = 190
	2 Tblsp = 25
Mushroom – canned	1 c = 120
	2 Tblsp = 15
Turkey – canned	1 c = 120
	2 Tblsp = 15
Green Giant Broccoli in Cheese Flavor Sauce	
	1 serving = 190
	1 c = 115
Grits – instant, all flavors	1 package = 95
Guinea Hen – roasted	1/2 = 250
Ham – various types	
Ham & Cheese loaf or roll	1 slice = 75
Ham & Cheese spread	1/4 c = 150
Ham salad spread	1/4 c = 130
Ham – chopped, canned	1 slice = 50
Ham – cured, w/average fat content	3 oz = 190
Ham – sliced	1 slice = 45
Healthy Choice meal choices	
Healthy Choice Beef Macaroni frozen entree	1 serving = 210
Healthy Choice Cacciatore Chicken, w/pasta & vegetables	1 serving = 265
Healthy Choice Chicken Enchilada Supreme w/rice, corn, dessert	1 serving = 300
Healthy Choice Chicken Teriyaki w/rice, mixed vegetables, dessert	1 serving = 270
Healthy Choice Country Roast Turkey w/gravy, rice	1 serving = 225

HEALTHY CHOICE – JENO'S PIZZA

Healthy Choice Mesquite Beef w/barbeque sauce, mashed potatoes, corn	1 serving = 320
Healthy Choice Mesquite Chicken Barbeque w/rice, mixed vegetables, dessert	1 serving = 310
Healthy Choice Salsbury Steak w/gravy, mashed potatoes, corn	1 serving = 325
Healthy Choice Spaghetti frozen entree	1 serving = 255
Healthy Choice Traditional Meat Loaf w/potatoes, vegetables, dessert	1 serving = 315
Healthy Choice Cheddar Broccoli Potatoes	1 serving = 330
Hearts of Palm – canned (basically zero)	0
Hominy – canned	1 c = 120
Honey	1 Tblsp = 65
Hormel – various products	
Hormel Canadian Style Bacon	1 slice = 70
Hormel Chili With Beans, Canned	1 c = 240
Hormel Chili, No Beans, Canned	1 c = 195
Hormel Corned Beef Hash, Canned	1 c = 385
Hormel Cure 81 Ham	1 slice = 90
Hormel Dinty Moore Beef Stew – canned	1 serving = 400
	1 c = 220
Hormel Pepperoni, Turkey	1 serving = 75
Hormel Roast Beef Hash, Canned	1 c = 385
Hormel Spam, Pork & Chicken	2 oz = 105
Hormel Spam, Pork And Ham	2oz = 175
Hormel Turkey Chili With Beans, Canned	1 c = 205
Hormel Vegetarian Chili With Beans, Canned	1 c = 205
Hormel Wrangler Beef Franks	1 = 160
Hot Pockets – various styles	
Hot Pockets Beef & Cheddar – frozen	1 serving = 405
Hot Pockets Croissant Pockets Chicken w/broccoli & cheese – frozen	1 serving = 300
Hot Pockets Ham 'n Cheese – frozen	1 serving = 340
Hot Pockets Pepperoni Pizza – frozen	1 serving = 365
Hummus	1/4 c = 170
Hush Puppies, Home Made	1 = 50
Ice Cream Cones – cake or wafer-type	1 = 15
Ice Cream Cones – sugar waffle, rolled-type	1 = 40
Ice Cream – French vanilla, soft-serve	1 c = 370
Ice Cream – vanilla, light, not soft-serve	1 c = 185
Ice Cream – vanilla, light, soft-serve	1 c = 220
Ice Cream – vanilla, regular	1 c = 290
Ice Cream – vanilla, rich	1 c = 515
Jack's Combination Sausage & Pepperoni Pizza – frozen	1 serving = 350
Jack's Original Pepperoni Pizza – frozen	1 serving = 325
Jams & Preserves	1 Tblsp = 55
Jellies	1 Tblsp = 55
Jeno's Combination Pizza, Sausage & Pepperoni – frozen	1 serving = 490

Jeno's Crisp 'n Tasty Pepperoni Pizza – frozen	1 serving = 515
Jimmy Dean Sausage Biscuits – frozen, pre-cooked	1 = 190
Kale, Boiled (basically zero)	0
Keebler Cookies – Chocolate Graham Selects	1 = 145
Keebler Cookies – Golden Vanilla Wafers	1 = 20
Kellogg's – various products	
Kellog's Eggo Waffles	1 = 70
Kellog's Lo Fat Pop Tarts – all	1 = 190
Kellog's Pop Tarts Swirls – all	1 = 255
Kellog's Pop Tarts – all	1 = 205
Ketchup (catsup) (basically zero)	0
Kielbasa	1 sausage = 85
	1 oz = 65
Kiwi Fruit – fresh	1 = 55
Knockwurst	1 = 220
Kraft Products – various types	
Kraft Breakstone's Fat Free Sour Cream	2 Tblsp = 30
Kraft Breakstone's Sour Cream	2 Tblsp = 30
Kraft Breyers Low-fat Strawberry Yogurt	1 container = 220
Kraft Cheese Singles, American Non-fat	1 slice = 30
Kraft Cheez Whiz Light	1 Tblsp = 40
Kraft Cheez Whiz Regular	1 Tblsp = 100
Kraft Country Time Lemonade Mix	1 c = 65
Kraft Foods – Shake 'n' Bake Original Recipe for Pork	1 serving = 105
Kraft Jell-o Brand Instant Pudding – home-cooked	1 serving = 110
Kraft Kool-Aid Special Soft Drink	1 serving = 115
Kraft Mayo Fat Free	1 Tblsp = 10
Kraft Mayo Light	1 Tblsp = 50
Kraft Miracle Whip Light	1 Tblsp = 35
Kraft Miracle Whip Non-fat	1 Tblsp = 15
Kraft Stove Top Stuffing Mix – Chicken Flavoror	1 serving = 105
Kraft Sugar Free Kool-Aid (basically zero)	0
Kraft Tang	1 c = 90
Kraft Velveeta	1 slice = 1 oz = 85
Kraft Velveeta Light	1 slice = 1 oz = 60
Kumquats, fresh (basically zero)	0
Lamb – various types	
Lamb leg – cooked (not fried)	4 oz = 290
Lamb loin – cooked (not fried)	4 oz = 355
Lamb rib – cooked (not fried)	4 oz meat = 385
Lamb shoulder – cooked (not fried)	4 oz = 405
Lard	1 Tblsp = 115
	1 cup = 1, 850
Lean Pockets Glazed Chicken Supreme (frozen)	1 serving = 235
Leeks – boiled (basically zero)	0
Lemon Juice (basically zero)	0
Lemon – fresh, whole or slices (basically zero)	0

Lettuce, fresh (basically zero)	0
Lime Juice (basically zero)	0
Lime – fresh, whole or slices (basically zero)	0
Lobster – cooked	4 oz = 110
Lobster, Spiny – cooked (not fried)	4 oz = 165
Loganberries – fresh frozen	1/2 c = 40
Louis Rich – various styles	
Louis Rich Chicken Breast	1 slice = 50
Louis Rich Franks	1 = 90
Louis Rich Sausage – turkey, smoked	1 serving = 90
Louis Rich Turkey Bacon	1 slice = 25
Louis Rich Turkey Bologna	1 slice = 50
Louis Rich Turkey Breast	1 slice = 50
Louis Rich Turkey Ham (10% water)	1 slice = 32
Louis Rich Turkey Nuggets/sticks (breaded)	1 piece = 75
Louis Rich Turkey Salami	1 serving = 40
Luncheon Meat, Beef	1 slice = 85
Luncheon Meat, Pork	1 slice = 70
Macaroni – home-cooked	1 c = 195
Mangos – fresh	1 = 135
Margarine – different types	
Margarine Spread, fat-free in tub	1/2 c = 50
	1 Tblsp = 5
Margarine Corn, hard or soft	1 c = 1 stick = 815
	1/2 c = 1/2 stick = 410
	1 tsp = 35
Margarine-like spread	1 c = 800
	1 tsp = 15
Marie Callender's Foods	
Beef Stroganoff w/carrots & peas	1 serving = 600
Marie Callender's Chicken & Potatoes Pie (frozen)	1 c = 500
Marie Callender's Escalloped Noodles	
& Chicken	1 serving = 397
Marie Callender's Turkey w/gravy & dressing,	
broccoli	1 serving = 504
Marmalade, Orange	1 Tblsp = 50
Melon Balls – frozen	1 c frozen = 60
Melons, Cantaloupe – fresh	1/4 = 75
Melons, Honeydew – fresh	1/4 = 60
Milk Shakes – thick chocolate or vanilla	1 c = 270
Milk – various types	
1%	1 c = 100
	1 Tblsp = 5
2%	1 c = 120
	1 Tblsp = 10
Buttermilk, low-fat	1 c = 100
	1 Tblsp = 5
Condensed, Sweetened (canned)	1/2 c = 490
	1 Tblsp = 60

MILK PRODUCTS – OAT CEREALS

Evaporated (canned, not diluted)	1/2 c = 170
	1 Tblsp = 20
Evaporated (canned, non-fat, not diluted)	1/2 c = 100
	1 Tblsp = 10
Chocolate	1 c = 210
Chocolate – low-fat	1 c = 160
Chocolate – hot cocoa (homemade)	1 c = 195
Goat	1 c = 170
Non-fat	1 c = 85
	1 Tblsp = 5
Soy	1 c = 80
Milk – Whole	1 c = 150
	1 Tblsp = 10
Molasses	1 Tblsp = 55
Muffins – various choices	
Blueberry – prebaked	1 small = 185
Blueberry – homemade	1 = 160
Corn – prebaked	1 = 200
Corn – homemade	1 = 180
English – all types	1 = 140
Plain – homemade	1 = 170
Mushrooms – boiled or fresh (basically zero)	0
Mussels – cooked (not fried)	4 oz = 195
Nabisco Crackers	
Nabisco Grahams Crackers	1 square = 15
Nabisco Ritz Crackers	1 = 15
Nabisco Wheat Thins Crackers	1 = 15
Nectarines – fresh	1 = 65
Nestea Ice Tea – Lemon Flavor	1 c = 90
Noodles – various types	
Chinese, Chow Mein	1 c = 235
Egg or Spinach – home-cooked	1 c = 215
Japanese	1 c = 115
Nuts – various types	
Almonds – honey-roasted	1/4 c = 215
Cashews – fresh	1/4 c = 200
Cashews – dry-roasted	1/4 c = 195
Chestnuts, Chinese – fresh or roasted	1 oz = 65
Hazelnuts or Filberts – fresh or dry-roasted	1/4 c = 45
Macadamia – fresh or dry-roasted	1/4 c = 240
Mixed Nuts – dry-roasted, w/peanuts	1/4 c = 205
Mixed Nuts – oil-roasted, w/peanuts	1/4 c = 220
Pine – dried	10 nuts = 5, 1 oz = 175
Pistachio – fresh or dry-roasted	1/4 c = 180
Walnuts – black or English	1 Tblsp = 50
Oat Bran – cooked	1 c = 90
Oat Cereals – various types	
Oatmeal – instant, bran & raisins	1 c = 160
Oatmeal – instant, w/cinnamon & spice	1 c = 265
Oatmeal – instant, w/raisins & spice	1 c = 245

OAT CEREALS – OSCAR MAYER

Oatmeal – Quaker Brown Sugar Bliss	1 c = 190
Oatmeal – Quaker Instant, all flavors	1 c = 135
Quaker Instant, Apples & Cinnamon	1 c = 125
Quaker Instant, Maple & Brown Sugar	1 c = 155
Quaker Quick 'n Hearty – all flavors	1 c = 165
Oatmeal – regular or quick or instant	1 c = 145
Oil for Cooking – various types	
Canola	1/2 c = 965
Coconut	1/2 c = 940
	1 Tblsp = 115
Corn	1/2 c = 965
Olive	1/2 c = 955
	1 Tblsp = 120
Peanut	1/2 c = 955
	1 Tblsp = 120
Sesame	1/2 c = 965
	1 Tblsp = 120
Soybean	1/2 c = 965
	1 Tblsp = 120
Sunflower	1/2 c = 965
	1 Tblsp = 120
Okra, Boiled (basically zero)	0
Old El Paso Chili w/beans – canned	1 serving = 250
Olives, Ripe, Canned	1/4 c = 40
Onions, fresh or cooked (basically zero)	0
Orange Juice – fresh or concentrate (made w/water)	1 c = 110
Orange-Grapefruit Juice –canned, unsweetened	1 c = 105
Oranges – fresh	1 = 85
Oscar Mayer – various products	
Oscar Mayer Bologna (beef, light)	1 slice = 55
Oscar Mayer Bologna (beef)	1 slice = 90
Oscar Mayer Bologna (fat-ree)	1 slice = 20
Oscar Mayer Chicken Breast (fat-free)	1 slice = 45
Oscar Mayer Chicken Breast (honey-glazed)	1 slice = 55
Oscar Mayer Ham & Cheese Loaf	1 slice = 65
Oscar Mayer Ham (fat-free, boiled, smoked, honey)	1 slice = 65
Oscar Mayer Chopped Ham	1 slice = 50
Oscar Mayer Luncheon Loaf (spiced)	1 slice = 65
Oscar Mayer Old-Fashioned Loaf	1 slice = 65
Oscar Mayer Olive Loaf	1 slice = 75
Oscar Mayer Pickle Pimiento Loaf	1 slice = 75
Oscar Mayer Salami	1 serving = 95
Oscar Mayer Sandwich Spread	1 serving = 70
Oscar Mayer Sausage Links	1 = 80
Oscar Mayer Sausage – Smokie Links	1 = 130
Oscar Mayer Smokies Sausage – little size	1 link = 30
Oscar Mayer Smokies, regular size	1serving = 130
Oscar Mayer Summer Sausage	1 slice = 140
Oscar Mayer Turkey Breast – fat-free	1 slice = 40

OSCAR MAYER – PEPPERS

Oscar Mayer Wiener – beef, fat-free	1 = 40
Oscar Mayer Wiener – beef, full bun length	1 = 185
Oscar Mayer Wiener – little	1 = 30
Oscar Mayer Wiener – pork, turkey & beef, regular length	1 = 145
Oscar Mayer Wiener – turkey & cheese	1 = 145
Oscar Meyer Wiener – light	1 = 110
Oysters	
Oysters – breaded & fried	6 = 175
Oysters – cooked (not fried)	6 = 60
Oysters – fresh	6 = 55
Pancakes – various types	
Buttermilk – homemade	1 = 85
Dry Mix – homecooked	1 = 75
Frozen – precooked	1 = 165
Homemade – from scratch	1 = 85
Potato – homemade	1 = 205
Papaya Nectar – canned	1 c = 145
Papayas – fresh	1/2 = 125
Passion-Fruit Juice – fresh	1 c = 135
Passion-Fruit – fresh (basically zero)	0
Pasta – homemade	1 c = 295
Pastrami	1 slice = 100
Pastrami – fat-free	6 slices = 55
Pastrami – turkey	1 slice = 40
Pate Goose Liver – smoked, canned	1 Tblsp = 60
Peach Nectar – canned	1 c = 135
Peaches – canned in heavy syrup	1 c = 195
Peaches – canned in light syrup	1 c = 135
Peaches – fresh	1 = 70
Peanut Butter – chunky or smooth	2 Tblsp = 190
Peanuts – boiled in-hull	1 c in shells = 200
Peanuts – shelled, fresh/oil-roasted/dry-roasted	1/4 c = 210
Pear Nectar – canned	1 c = 150
Pears – canned in heavy syrup	1 c = 195
Pears – canned in light syrup	1 c = 145
Pears – fresh	1 = 125
Peas & Carrots – canned	1 c = 95
Peas – Green, cooked	1 c = 135
Pecans – fresh or dry-roasted	1/4 c = 210
Pepperidge Farm Apple Turnovers – frozen, home-baked	1 = 285
Pepperidge Farm Crusty Italian Bread, Garlic	1 slice = 185
Pepperoni	1 slice = 25
Pepperoni pizza – frozen	1 serving = 400
Peppers – various types	
Banana – uncooked (basically zero)	0
Chili, green – canned (basically zero)	0
Jalapeno – fresh or cooked (basically zero)	0
Sweet green or red – fresh or cooked (basically zero)	0

PERSIMMON – POMEGRANATES

Persimmon – fresh	1 = 30
Pheasant – roasted	1 = 800
Phyllo Dough	1 sheet = 55
Pickle & Pimiento Loaf	1 slice = 75
Pickle Relish – sweet (basically zero)	0
Pickle – cucumber, sweet (basically zero)	0
Pickle – cucumber, dill (basically zero)	0
Pie Crust – various type	
Graham Cracker – homemade	1 whole shell = 1,035
Standard-type – dry mix, home-baked	1 whole shell = 800
Standard-type – frozen, home-baked	1 whole shell = 650
Standard-type – homemade	1 whole shell = 950
Pie – various types	
Apple – premade	1 piece = 295
Apple – homemade	1 piece = 410
Banana Cream – homemade	1 piece = 255
Banana Cream – no-bake mix, home-baked	1 piece = 230
Blueberry – premade	1 piece = 290
Blueberry – premade	1 piece = 360
Cherry – premade	1 piece = 325
Cherry – homemade	1 piece = 485
Chocolate Cream – premade	1 piece = 300
Chocolate Mousse – no-bake mix, home-baked	1 piece = 245
Coconut Cream – no-bake mix, home-baked	1 piece = 260
Coconut Cream – premade	1 piece = 190
Coconut Custard – premade	1 piece = 270
Egg Custard – premade	1 piece = 220
Fried Fruit Pie	1 pie = 405
Lemon Meringue – premade	1 piece = 305
Lemon Meringue – homemade	1 piece = 360
Peach	1 piece = 260
Pecan – premade	1 piece = 450
Pecan – homemade	1 piece = 505
Pumpkin – premade	1 piece = 230
Pumpkin – homemade	1 piece = 315
Pimento – canned (basically zero)	0
Pineapple juice – canned, unsweetened	1 c = 140
Pineapple juice – from frozen concentrate	
unsweetened, made w/water	1 c = 130
Pineapple slices – canned in juice	1 slice = 30
Pineapple slices – canned in heavy syrup	1 slice = 40
Pineapple – fresh	1 c diced = 75
Plantains – cooked	1/2 c = 90
Plantains – fresh	1 = 220
Plums, purple – canned in juice	1 = 25, 1 c = 145
Plums, purple – canned in heavy syrup	1 = 41, 1 c = 230
Plum – fresh	1 = 35
Polaner All-Fruit Strawberry Spread	1 Tblsp = 40
Polish Sausage	1 = 740
Pomegranates – fresh	1 = 105

POPCORN – RASPBERRIES

Popcorn – air-popped	2 c = 60
Popcorn – cheese-flavored	2 c = 115
Popcorn – oil-popped	2 c = 110
Pork Sausage	1 link = 50, 1 patty = 100
Pork Skins – plain	2 c = 310
Pork Chops – center cut, cooked (not fried)	1 = 200
Pork Chops -- center cut, cooked (pan-fried)	1 = 215
Pork – country-style ribs	3 oz meat = 280
Pork – tenderloin, cooked	3 oz = 140
Pork Loin – cooked	3 oz = 210
Pork Spareribs – cooked	3 oz meat = 335
Potato Chips – all types	10 = 85
Potato Salad – homemade	1 c = 360
Potato Sticks	1 c = 190
Potato, Baked	1 large = 280
Potatoes Au Gratin – dry mix, made w/milk & water	1 c = 225
Potatoes Au Gratin – homemade	1 c = 325
Potatoes – boiled	1 = 120
Potatoes – canned, hhite	1 = 20
Potatoes – French Fried, frozen, home-fried	20 strips = 200
Potatoes – hash brown, frozen, home-fried	1 c = 340
Potatoes – mashed, from flakes, made w/milk	1 c = 165
Potatoes – mashed, homemade w/milk	1 c = 160
Potatoes O'Brien – homemade	1 c = 155
Potatoes – scalloped, dry mix, made w/milk & water	1 c = 230
Pretzels – hard	1 small twist = 30
Prune juice – canned	1/2 c = 90
Prunes – canned in heavy syrup	1/2 c = 125
Prunes – cooked w/sugar	1/2 c = 155
Puddings – various styles	
Pudding – banana, premade, canned	1 c = 290
Pudding – chocolate or coconut, dry mix, homecooked w/milk	1 c = 325
Pudding – chocolate, premade	1 can = 190
Pudding – coconut cream, dry mix, homecooked w/milk	1 c = 290
Pudding – lemon, premade	1 c = 280
Pudding – lemon, dry mix, home-cooked w/milk	1 c = 340
Pudding – rice, premade	1 c = 370
Pudding – tapioca, premade	1 c = 270
Pudding – vanilla, premade	1 c = 295
Pudding – vanilla, dry mix, home-cooked w/milk	1 c = 325
Puff Pastry – frozen, homebaked	1 shell = 260
Pumpkin – canned	1 c = 85
Quail – roasted	1 = 110
Radicchio – fresh (basically zero)	0
Radishes – fresh (basically zero)	0
Raisins, All Types	1/2 c = 215
Raspberries – canned in heavy syrup	1/2 c = 115
Raspberries – frozen, sweetened	1/2 c frozen = 130

RASPBERRIES – SAUCES

Raspberries – fresh	1/2 c = 30
Red Baron Pizza – various types	
Red Baron Pepperoni Pizza – frozen	1 serving = 440
Red Baron Premium Deep Dish Singles Pizza	
– pepperoni	1 serving = 480
Red Baron Special Deluxe Pizza	1 serving = 335
Red Baron Supreme Pizza – sausage,	
mushroom,pepperoni	1 serving = 345
Rhubarb – fresh	1 stalk = 10
	1 c diced = 25
Rice Bar – chocolate chip	1 = 115
Rice Cakes	1 = 35
Rice Noodles – home-cooked	1 c = 190
Rice, Brown – cooked	1 c = 215
Rice, White – cooked	1 c = 205
Rolls – various types	
Dinner – prebaked	1 = 130
Dinner – homemade	1 = 135
Hamburger or Hotdog	1 = 125
Hard	1 = 165
Rutabagas – boiled	1 c cubed = 65
Salad Dressings – various types	
French	2 Tblsp = 135
French – diet, low-calorie	1 Tblsp = 20
Italian	2 Tblsp = 140
Italian – diet	1 Tblsp = 15
Kraft Fat-Free Italian	2 Tblsp = 20
Kraft Fat-Free Ranch	2 Tblsp = 50
Kraft Italian	2 Tblsp = 55
Kraft Light Ranch	2 Tblsp = 75
Kraft Ranch	2 Tblsp = 150
Kraft Zesty Italian	2 Tblsp = 110
Russian	1 Tblsp = 75
Russian – low-calorie	1 Tblsp = 25
Sesame Seed	1 Tblsp = 70
Thousand Island	1 Tblsp = 60
Thousand Island – diet, low-calorie	1 Tblsp = 25
Vinegar & Oil	2 Tblsp = 140
Salad, Tuna	1 c = 385
Salami	1 slice = 70
	1 oz = 120
Sauces – different types	
Barbecue	3 Tblsp = 35
Kraft Barbecue – Original & Hickory Smoke	2 Tblsp = 40
Nestle Stir Fry	1 package = 2175
Nestle Sweet N' Sour	1 package = 2490
Nestle Teriyaki	1 package = 2690
Plum	3 Tblsp = 105
Prego 100% Natural Spaghetti	1/2 c = 545
Ragu Old World Style Smooth Pasta	1/2 c = 80

Sauerkraut – canned (basically zero)	0
Sausage & Pepperoni Pizza – frozen	1 serving = 385
Sausage – various types	
Italian	1 link = 215
Polish	1 oz = 90
Turkey Links	1 link = 65
Smoked Link	1 little link = 55
Turkey – regular & Italian	1 oz = 45
Scallop – breaded & fried	1 = 35
Semolina	1 c = 600
Sesame Seeds – whole, dried	1 Tblsp = 50
Shallots – freeze-dried	1/2 c = 25
Sherbet – orange	1 c = 205
Shrimp – breaded & fried	4 large = 75
Shrimp – cooked (not fried)	4 large = 22
Soups – various types	
Bean w/frankfurters – canned	1 c mixed w/water = 190
Bean w/pork – canned	1 c mixed w/water = 170
Beef Mushroom – canned	1 c mixed w/water = 75
Beef Noodle – canned	1 c mixed w/water = 85
Black Bean – canned	1 c mixed w/water = 115
Cheese – canned	1 c mixed w/milk = 230
	w/water = 155
Chicken Broth – canned	1 c mixed w/water = 40
Chicken Gumbo – canned	1 c mixed w/water = 55
Chicken Mushroom – canned	1 c mixed w/water = 130
Chicken Noodle – canned	1 c mixed w/water = 75
Chicken Vegetables – canned	1 c mixed w/water = 75
Chicken w/dumplings – canned	1 c mixed w/water = 95
Chicken w/rice – canned	1 c mixed w/water = 60
Chili Beef – canned	1 c mixed w/water = 170
Cream of Asparagus – canned	1 c mixed w/water = 85
Cream of Celery – canned	1 c mixed w/milk = 165
	w/water = 90
Cream of Chicken – canned	1 c mixed w/milk = 190
	w/water = 115
Cream of Mushroom – canned	1 c mixed w/milk = 205
	w/water = 130
Cream of Potato – canned	1 c mixed w/milk = 150
	1 c mixed w/water = 75
Lipton Cup-a-Soup – Broccoli & Cheese,	1 serving = 65
Lipton Cup-a-Soup	
– Chicken-Flavored Vegetables	1 serving = 50
Lipton Cup-a-Soup – Chicken Noodle w/meat	1 serving = 380
Lipton Cup-a-Soup – Cream of Chicken	1 serving = 70
Lipton Cup-a-Soup – Cream of Mushroom	1 serving = 60
Lipton Cup-a-Soup – Green Pea	1 serving = 75
Lipton Cup-a-Soup – Hearty Chicken Noodle	1 serving = 60
Lipton Cup-a-Soup – Hearty Chicken Supreme	1 serving = 90
Lipton Cup-a-Soup – Ring Noodle	1 serving = 55

SOUPS – SQUID

Lipton Cup-a-Soup – Spring Vegetables	1 serving = 45
Lipton Cup-a-Soup – Tomato	1 serving = 95
Lipton Fat-Free Cup-a-Soup Chicken & Pasta	1 serving = 45
Lipton Fat-Free Cup-a-Soup Chicken Broth	1 serving = 20
Lipton Kettle Creations – Chicken w/pasta & bean	1 serving = 105
Lipton Kettle Creations – Homestyle Lentil	1 serving = 125
Minestrone – canned	1 c mixed w/water = 80
Mushroom Barley – canned	1 c mixed w/water = 75
Mushroom w/beef stock – canned	1 c mixed w/water = 85
Onion – canned	1 c mixed w/water = 60
Pea, Green – canned	1 c mixed w/milk = 165
	w/water = 90

Soup

Pea, Green – canned	1 c mixed w/water = 165
Pea, Split w/ham – canned	1 c mixed w/water = 190
Progresso Beef Barley	1 c = 140
Progresso Chicken Noodle	1 c = 75
Progresso Chicken Rice w/vegetables	1 c = 90
Progresso Garlic & Pasta	1 c = 100
Progresso Lentil	1 c = 125, 2 Tblsp = 15
Progresso Minestrone	1 c = 125, 2 Tblsp = 15
Progresso Split Pea	1 c = 180
Progresso Tomato Garden	1 c = 90
Progresso Vegetables	1 c = 800, 1 tsp = 15
Progresso, Cream of Broccoli	1 c = 90
Tomato Beef w/noodle – canned	1 c mixed w/water = 140
Tomato Bisque – canned	1 c mixed w/milk = 200
	w/water = 125
Tomato Rice – canned	1 c mixed w/water = 120
Tomato – canned	1 c mixed w/milk = 160
	w/water = 85
Turkey Noodle – canned	1 c mixed w/water = 70
Turkey Vegetable – canned	1 c mixed w/water = 70
Vegetable Beef	1 c mixed w/water = 80
Vegetables w/beef broth – canned	1 c mixed w/water = 80
Vegetarian Vegetable – canned	1 c mixed w/water = 70
Soy Milk	1 c = 80
Soybeans, Green – boiled	1 c = 255
Spaghetti egg noodles – cooked	1 c = 195
Spaghetti, whole-wheat or spinach noodles – cooked	1 c = 180
Spinach Souffle – homemade	1 c = 220
Spinach – boiled (basically zero)	0
Spinach – fresh (basically zero)	0
Squash – different types	
Acorn or Hubbard – baked	1 c = 110
Butternut – baked	1 c = 80
Crooked, Straight, or Zucchini – boiled	1 c = 35
Spaghetti – boiled	1 c = 40
Squid, Fried	4 oz = 200

Stouffer's packaged foods – various items	
Stouffer's Chicken Enchilada & Mexican Rice	1 serving = 375
Stouffer's Chicken Pie – frozen	1 serving = 570
Stouffer's Creamed Chipped Beef	1 serving = 175
Stouffer's Creamed Spinach	1 serving = 1 c = 340
Stouffer's Delux French Bread Pizza	
– w/sausage, pepperoni & mushrooms	1 serving = 430
Stouffer's Escalloped Chicken & Noodles	1 serving = 420
Stouffer's French Bread Pizza	
– w/sausage & pepperoni	1 serving = 450
Stouffer's Lasagna w/meat & sausage	
– frozen entree	1 serving = 275
Stouffer's Lean Chicken A L'orange	
– w/sausage, broccoli & rice	1 serving = 270
Stouffer's Lean Cuisine Beef Potatoes Roast	
– w/whipped potatoes	1 serving = 205
Stouffer's Lean Cuisine Chicken & Vegetables	
– w/vermicelli	1 serving = 250
Stouffer's Lean Cuisine Chicken Enchilida	
– w/rice	1 serving = 300
Stouffer's Lean Cuisine Macaroni & Beef	
– in tomato sauce	1 serving = 250
Stouffer's Lean Cuisine Oriental Beef	
– w/vegetables & rice	1 serving = 240
Stouffer's Lean Cuisine Spaghetti	
– w/meat sauce	1 serving = 315
Stouffer's Lean Cuisine Spaghetti	
– w/meatballs & sauce	1 serving = 300
Stouffer's Lean Cuisine Stuffed Cabbage	
– w/meat, tomatoes, sauce, potatoes	1 serving = 200
Stouffer's Lean Cuisine Swedish Meatballs	
– w/pasta	1 serving = 275
Stouffer's Lean Lunch Express Rice &	
Chicken Stir-fry	1 serving = 270
Stouffer's Lunch Express Chicken Alfredo	
Fetuccini & Vegetables	1 serving = 375
Stouffer's Salsbury Steak, Gravy	
and Macroni & Cheese,	1 serving = 385
Stouffer's Stuffed Peppers w/beef	
in tomato sauce	1 serving = 190
Strawberries – canned in heavy syrup	1 c = 235
Strawberries – frozen, sweetened	1 c thawed = 200
Strawberries – frozen, unsweetened	1 c thawed = 75
Strawberries – fresh	1 c = 45
Strudel, Apple	1 piece = 195
Stuffing, Cornbread – homemade	1 c = 360
Succotash (corn & lima beans) – boiled	1 c = 220
Sugar – brown	1 Tblsp = 50
Sugar – granulated	1 tsp = 15
Sugar – powdered	1 tsp = 10

SUNFLOWER SEEDS – TOTINO'S PIZZA

Sunflower Seed Kernels – dry roasted	1/4 c = 185
Sunflower Seed Kernels – oil-roasted or toasted	1/4 c = 205
Sweet Rolls, Cinnamon – prebaked	1 large = 310
Sweet Rolls, Cinnamon – refrigerated dough w/frosting – homebaked	1 piece = 110
Sweetpotatoes – baked	1 large = 185
Sweetpotatoes, Candied – homemade	1 c = 285
Sweetpotatoes – canned in syrup	1 c = 340
Syrup, Corn – dark or light	1 c = 925
	1 Tblsp = 55
Syrup, Maple	3 Tblsp = 105
Syrup, Sorghum	3 Tblsp = 185
Syrup, Table Blends for pancakes	4 Tblsp = 230
Taco Shells, Baked	1 large = 100
Tangerine Juice – fresh or concentrate made w/water	1 c = 110
Tangerine – fresh	1 = 45
The Budget Gourmet Italian Sausage Lasagna	1 serving = 455
The Budget Gourmet Spinach Au Gratin	1 serving = 220
Toaster Pastries – all	1 = 205
Tofu – firm or soft	1 c = 75
Tomato juice – canned	1 c = 40
Tomato, Sauce – canned	1 c = 75
Tomatoes, Green or Ripe, fresh, cooked, or canned	1 large = 45
Tomatoes – sun-dried	1/2 c = 70
Tomatoes – sun-dried, packed in oil	1/2 c = 115
Tombstone Pizza – various types	
Tombstone Original Pepperoni Pizza – frozen, 12 Inch	1 serving = 315
Tombstone Original Pepperoni Pizza – frozen, 9 Inch	1 serving = 415
Tombstone Original Sausage & Mushroom Pizza – frozen	1 serving = 305
Tombstone Original Sausage & Pepperoni Pizza – frozen	1 serving = 330
Tony's Pizza – various types	
Tony's D'Primo Deep Dish Sausage Pizza	1 serving = 390
Tony's Pepperoni Pizza w/Italian Crust	1 serving = 405
Tony's Sausage & Pepperoni Pizza w/Italian Crust	1 serving = 435
Tony's Supreme Pizza w/everything	1 serving = 400
Tony's Taco Style Pizza	1 serving = 435
Toppings, Butterscotch Or Caramel	3 Tblsp = 355
Toppings, Pineapple	3 Tblsp = 160
Tortilla Chips, All Flavors	10 = 120
Tortillas, Corn – homemade	1 = 55
Tortillas, Flour – homemade	1 = 100
Tostada w/guacamole	1 = 180
Totino's Party Pizza Combination Sausage & Pepperoni – frozen	1 serving = 385
Totino's Party Pizza Pepperoni – frozen	1 serving = 365

Totino's Pizza Rolls Pizza Snacks, Hamburger – frozen	1 serving = 230
Totino's Pizza Snacks – pepperoni	1 serving = 385
Trail Mix – regular	1 c = 695
Trail Mix– tropical	1 c = 570
Trail Mix – w/chocolate chips, nuts & seeds	1 c = 705
Turkey & Potatoe Pie – frozen entrée	1 serving = 700
Turkey – breast meat	1 slice = 25
Turkey Ham	1 oz = 35, 1 slice = 40
Turkey Breast – fat-free, packaged	1 slice = 25
Turkey Roasted – 1/4 breast	meat w/skin = 265
	meat only = 205
Turkey Roasted – drumstick	meat w/skin = 190
	meat only = 160
Turkey Roasted – thigh	meat w/skin = 230
	meat only = 195
Turkey Roasted – wing	meat w/skin = 185
	meat only = 100
Turnip Greens – boiled (basically zero)	0
Turnip Root – boiled (basically zero)	0
Tyson brand foods	
Tyson Beef Stir Fry Kit w/rice, vegetables beef strips, sauce	1 serving = 435
Tyson Chicken Fajita Kit	1 serving = 130
Tyson Chicken Mesquite w/barbeque sauce, corn, potatoes	1 serving = 320
Tyson Roasted Chicken w/garlic sauce, pasta & vegetable medley	1 serving = 215
Veal – assorted cuts	
Veal Leg – breaded & fried	4 oz = 260
Veal Leg – cooked (not fried)	4 oz = 165
Veal Leg – fried (not breaded)	4 oz = 240
Veal Loin – cooked (not fried)	4 oz = 280
Veal Rib – cooked (not fried)	4 oz meat = 285
Veal Shoulder – cooked (not fried)	4 oz = 240
Vegetable Juice Cocktail	1 c = 45
Vegetables – mixed, canned or frozen, home-cooked	1 c = 85
Vienna Sausage	1 = 45
Waffles – assorted types	
Waffles – frozen, home-cooked	1 = 100
Waffles – homemade	1 = 220
Water chestnuts – canned	1/2 c slices = 35
	4 whole = 15
Watermelon – fresh	1 c = 60
Wild Rice – cooked	1 c = 165
Yogurts – assorted styles	
No Fruit, w/low-fat or skim milk	1 c = 190
No Fruit, w/whole milk	1 c = 190
Fruit w/low-fat or skim Milk	1 c = 250
Soft-serve frozen dessert – vanilla or chocolate	1 c = 230

A&W

Sandwiches	Calories
Cheeseburger	480
Crispy Chicken	580
Deluxe Bacon Cheeseburger	570
Deluxe Bacon Double Cheeseburger	880
Deluxe Cheeseburger	510
Deluxe Double Cheeseburger	790
Deluxe Hamburger	470
Grilled Chicken	280
Hamburger	440
Jr. Cheeseburger	490
Jr. Hamburger	430
Hot Dogs	
Cheese Dog	320
Chili Cheese Dog	350
Chili Dog (Coney)	310
Plain	280
Sides	
Fries w/ Cheese	350
Fries w/ Chili	370
Fries w/ Chili & Cheese	400
Fries, Large	430
Fries, Small	310
Onion Rings	350
Specialty Drinks	
A&W Root Beer – Diet	0
A&W Root Beer – Regular	110

Applebee's

Specialty Item	Calories
Bikini Banana Low Fat Strawberry Shortcake	230
Low Fat & Fabulous Brownie Sundae	325
Low Fat Asian Chicken Salad	715
Low Fat Blackened Chicken Salad	500
Low Fat Chicken Quesadilla	740
Low Fat Chicken Roma Rollup	640
Low Fat Garlic Chicken Pasta	530
Low Fat Grilled Chicken Pasta	875
Low Fat Veggie Quesadilla	595
Low Fat Whitefish w/Mango Salsa	440

Arby's

Roast Beef Sandwiches	Calories
Arby-Q®	360
Arby's Melt w/Cheddar	340
Beef 'N Cheddar	480
Big Montana®	630

ARBY'S

Giant Roast Beef	480
Junior Roast Beef	310
Regular Roast Beef	350
Super Roast Beef	470
Other Sandwiches	
Chicken Bacon 'N Swiss	610
Chicken Breast Fillet	540
Chicken Cordon Bleu	630
Grilled Chicken Deluxe	450
Hot Ham 'N Swiss	340
Roast Chicken Club	520
Sub Sandwiches	
French Dip	440
Hot Ham 'N Swiss	530
Italian	780
Philly Beef 'N Swiss	700
Roast Beef	760
Turkey	630
Market Fresh Sandwiches	
Market Fresh Ultimate BLT	820
Roast Beef & Swiss	810
Roast Chicken Caesar	820
Roast Ham & Swiss	730
Roast Turkey & Swiss	760
Roast Turkey Ranch & Bacon	880
Market Fresh Salads (No Dressing)	
Caesar Salad	90
Caesar Side Salad	45
Chicken Finger Salad	570
Grilled Chicken Caesar	230
Turkey Club Salad	350
Light Menu	
Light Grilled Chicken	280
Light Roast Chicken Deluxe	260
Light Roast Turkey Deluxe	260
Salads	
Garden	70
Grilled Chicken	210
Roast Chicken	160
Side	25
Side Items & Snacks	
Baked Potato Deluxe	650
Baked Potato w/Broccoli 'N Cheddar	540
Baked Potato w/Butter &Sour Cream	500
Cheddar Curly Fries	460
Chicken Finger Snack w/curly Fries	580
Chicken Finger 4-Pack	640
Curly Fries Large	620
Curly Fries Med	400
Curly Fries Small	310

ARBY'S

Homestyle Fries Child-size	220
Homestyle Fries Large	560
Homestyle Fries Med	370
Homestyle Fries Small	300
Jalapeno Bites™	330
Mozzarella Sticks (4)	470
Onion Petals	410
Potato Cakes (2)	250
Desserts	
Apple Turnover (w/icing)	420
Cherry Turnover (w/icing)	410
Breakfast Items	
Add Egg	110
Add Slice Swiss Cheese	45
Biscuit w/Butter	280
Biscuit w/Bacon	320
Biscuit w/Ham	330
Biscuit w/Sausage	440
Croissant w/Bacon	300
Croissant w/Ham	310
Croissant w/Sausage	420
French Toastix (No Syrup)	370
Sourdough w/Bacon	380
Sourdough w/Ham	220
Sourdough w/Sausage	330
Condiments	
Arby's Sauce® Pack	15
Au Jus Sauce	5
BBQ Dipping Sauce	40
BBQ Vinaigrette Dressing	140
Bleu Cheese Dressing	300
Bronco Berry Sauce™	90
Buttermilk Ranch Dressing	360
Buttermilk Ranch Dressing Reduced Cal.	60
Caesar Dressing	310
Croutons, Cheese & Garlic	100
Croutons, Seasoned	30
French Toast Syrup	130
German Mustard Pack	5
Honey French Dressing	290
Honey Mustard Sauce	130
Horsey Sauce® Pack	60
Italian Dressing, Reduced Calorie	25
Italian Parmesan Dressing	240
Ketchup Pack	10
Marinara Sauce	35
Mayonnaise Pack	90
Mayonnaise Pack Light, Cholesterol-Free	20
Tangy Southwest Sauce™	250
Thousand Island Dressing	290

Beverages

Chocolate Shake	480
Hot Chocolate	110
Jamocha Shake	470
Milk	120
Orange Juice	140
Strawberry Shake	500
Vanilla Shake	470

Au Bon Pain

Breakfast Items	**Calories**
Cholesterol & Fat-free Egg	25
Egg & Bagel w/Cheese & Bacon	560
Egg & Bagel w/Cheese Or Bacon	480
Egg & Bagel	400

Bagels

Asiago Cheese	380
Cinnamon Crisp	430
Cinnamon Raisin	330
Dutch Apple	470
Everything	330
French Toast	420
Honey 9 Nine	360
Jalapeno Cheddar	290
Plain	300
Sesame Seed	340

Croissants

Almond	510
Apple	220
Chocolate	380
Cinnamon Raisin	340
Ham & Cheese	330
Plain	250
Raspberry	340
Spinach & Cheese	250
Sweet Cheese	350

Scones

Asiago Cheese	430
Cinnamon	480
Orange w/icing	410

Muffins

Apple Spice	510
Banana Walnut	560
Blueberry	480
Carrot Walnut Spice	550
Corn	440
Cranberry Nut	540
Double Chocolate	540
Low Fat Chocolate Cake	320
Low Fat Triple Berry	290

AU BON PAIN

Pumpkin	540
Raisin Bran	520

Cookies

Chocolate Chip	260
Chocolate Chunk Macadamia	290
Chocolate Dipped Cranberry Almond Macaroon	320
Chocolate Dipped Shortbread	300
Double Chocolate	340
English Toffee	200
GingerBread Man	270
Oatmeal Raisin	240
Peanut Butter Chunk	270
Shortbread	270
Walnut Raisin	280
White Chocolate Dipped Chocolate Shortbread	380

Dessert Bars

Apple Crumb Cake	540
Blond w/Nuts	570
Butter Crumb Cake	790
Cheescake Brownie	470
Chocolate Chip Brownie	480
Pecan Brownie	510
Raspberry Crumb Cake	770
Rocky Road Brownie	550

Strudels & Danishes

Apple	410
Cherry	390
Cranberry	370
Lemon	390
Sweet Cheese	430

Special Delights

Cinnamon Roll	320
Crème De Fluer	550
Pecan Roll	750
Oatmeal Bar	150

Bread & Rolls

Apple Spice Loaf	860
Asiago Flat Bread	330
Baguette	120
Braided Roll	420
Bread Bowl	640
Country White Sandwich Loaf	110
Ficelle	500
Focaccia	740
Four Grain	310
Hearth Roll	240
Lavash	250
Multigrain Loaf	130
Parisienne	120
Petite Pain	200

AU BON PAIN

Rosemary Garlic Bread Stick	200
Three Seed Sandwich Roll	330
Tomato Herb Loaf	140

Cream Cheese Spreads (2 oz serving)

Veggie Or Walnut	140
Plain	120
Sun Dried Tomato	70

Sandwiches

Arizona	580
Chicken	740
Chicken & Mozzarella Focaccia	800
Chicken Tarragon w/Field Greens	630
Honey Dijon Chicken	630
Mozzarella, Tomato, & Pesto	820
Smoked Turkey Club	760
Thai Chicken	490
Chicken, Ham, Cambozola	1140
Roast Beef & Pepperoncini	1160
Turkey, Ham, Provolone	1030

Wraps

Chicken Caesar	600
Fields And Feta	570
Honey Smoked Turkey	540
Southwestern Tuna	690
Mediterranean	560

Sandwich Fillings

Brie Cheese	150
Cambozola Cheese	200
Cheddar Cheese	170
Chicken Breast	120
Chicken Tarragon	210
Ham	150
Hummus	100
Lavash	250
Provolone Cheese	140
Roast Beef	150
Swiss Cheese	160
Tuna Salad Mix	170
Turkey Breast	120

Salads

Caesar	240
Charbroiled Salmon Filet, Yellow Peppers	210
Chef	290
Chicken Caesar	310
Cobb	460
Garden	160
Mediterranean Chicken	230
Mozzarella & Red Pepper	360
Nicoise	350
Side Garden	90

Thai Chicken	260
Tomato, Mozzarella w/Basil Pesto	280
Tuna Salad	430

Salad Dressings (2 Tblsp)

Balsamic Vinaigrette	190
Blue Cheese	130
Caesar	160
Fat-free Raspberry	35
Lite Honey Mustard	100
Lite Olive Oil Vinaigrette	60
Lite Ranch	110
Mediterranean	80
Parmesan & Peppercorn	170
Thai Peanut	70

Soups & Stews (8 oz)

Autumn Pumpkin	140
Baked Stuffed Potato	240
Beef	210
Black Bean	170
Broccoli Cheddar	230
Chicken Chili	210
Chicken Florentine	170
Chicken Noodle	90
Chicken Stew	230
Clam Chowder	220
Classic Chili w/beans	190
Corn & Green Chili Bisque	160
Corn Chowder	240
Curried Rice And Lentil	100
French Moroccan Tomato Lentil	110
French Onion	80
Garden Vegetable	40
Lobster Bisque	250
Mediterranean Pepper	190
Mediterranean Seafood	170
Old Fashioned Tomato	130
Pasta E Fagiolo	160
Potato Cheese	180
Potato Leek	190
Red Beans, Rice, & Sausage	180
Southern Black eyed Pea	190
Southwest Tortilla Soup	140
Southwest Vegetable	150
Split Pea	140
Tomato Florentine	70
Turkey Chili	200
Tuscan Vegetable	130
Vegetable Beef Barley	80
Vegetarian Chili	170
Vegetarian Lentil	110

Vegetarian Minestrone	70
Wild Mushroom Bisque	110
Specialty Drinks	
Apple Cider	250
Frozen Mocha Blast	270
Iced Cappuccino (Reg)	220
Mocha Blast (Reg)	351

Atlanta Bread Company

Bagels (4 oz.)	**Calories**
Asiago	350
Banana	350
Blueberry	340
Chocolate Chip	330
Cinnamon Raisin	340
Everything	310
Honey Wheat	330
Jalapeno	330
Onion	300
Plain	340
Poppy Seed	310
Pumpernickel	300
Sesame Seed	310
Breads (2 oz.)	
Asiago	150
Braided Challah	150
Chocolate Raisin Bread	200
Cinnamon Raisin	170
Cracked Wheat	160
Focaccia	170
French	140
Honey Wheat	150
Nine Grain	150
Olive	180
Onion	160
Pecan Raisin Loaf	200
Pesto	150
PowerLoaf MultiLoaf	150
Pumpernickel	150
Rosemary Focaccia	190
Rye	150
Sourdough	140
Sun Dried Tomato	150
Tuscana Parmesan	160
Rolls (2.6 oz.)	
French	180
Sourdough	190
Muffins (4 oz.)	
Apple Cinnamon	400
Banana Walnut	440

ATLANTA BREAD CO.

Blueberry	430
Chocolate Chip	460
Chocolate Mocha	470
Cranberry Apple	390
Cranberry Orange Walnut	440
Honey Raisin Bran	460
Lemon Poppy Seed	460
Low Fat Apple Cinnamon	310
Low Fat Banana	310
Low Fat Blueberry	310
Low Fat Chocolate	340
Low Fat Pumpkin	290
Peaches/Crème	530
Pumpkin	370
Zucchini	480
Muffin Tops (3 oz.)	
Banana Walnut	330
Blueberry	320
Chocolate Chip	340
Chocolate Mocha	350
Pumpkin	280
Salads	
Caesar Salad	220
Chicken Caesar	310
Chicken Curry	340
Chicken House	115
Chicken Salad	310
Chopstix Chicken	470
Fruit	140
Greek	120
Greek Chicken	210
House	35
Tuna	240
Sandwiches	
ABC Special®	510
Avocado	630
Bella Basil Chicken Sandwich	780
CharGrilled Chicken Pesto Panini	740
Chicken Curry	630
Chicken Salad	600
Cordon Bleu Panini	590
Cuban Pork Loin Panini	740
Honey Maple Ham	420
Italian Vegetarian Panini	610
Pastrami	440
Roast Beef	450
Tuna	530
Turkey Breast	420
Turkey Club Panini	780
Veggie	290

ATLANTA BREAD CO.

Soups (1 Cup)

Baked Potato	210
Black Bean & Rice	110
Black Bean w/ Ham	200
Chicken Chili	220
Chicken Gumbo	110
Chicken 'n Dumpling	240
Chicken Noodle	110
Chicken Tortilla	140
Chili w/ Beans	280
Clam Chowder	270
Country Bean	140
Cream of Broccoli	150
French Onion	60
Garden Veggie	80
Italian Style Wedding	120
Lentil & Roasted Garlic	200
Mushroom Barley & Sage	75
Pasta Fagioli	160
Seven Bean w/ Ham	240
Southwest Chicken	180
Szechuan Hot & Sour	80
Tomato Florentine	120
Tomato, Fennel & Dill	100
Vegetable Chili	180
Wisconsin Cheese	210

Specialty Sweets (1)

Austrian Pretzel	520
Bear Claw	520
Brownies	500
Chocolate Macadamia Biscotti	140
Cinnamon Nut Raisin Rolls	800
Cinnamon Rolls	650
Cinnamon Scone	340
Cranberry Scone	280
Eclairs	140
Key Lime Pie	450
Lemon Scone	340
Maple Oat Walnut Scone	360
Raspberry Scone	360
Sticky Bun	490
Vanilla Almond Biscotti	130

Cream Cheeses (2 oz.)

Chive	190
Honey Walnut Raisin	200
Olive	180
Raspberry	180
Veggie	190

Smoothies (16 oz.)

Heath Coffee	235

ATLANTA BREAD CO.

Kona Mocha Coffee	235
Pineapple Mango Banana	220
Spiced Chai Tea	130
Strawberry Banana	250
Strawberry Banana Blueberry	240
Vanilla Cafechillo	235
Croissants (1)	
Almond	580
Apple Filled	380
Butter	300
Cheese Filled	460
Chocolate	600
Raspberry Cheese	420
Danish (1)	
Apple	600
Blueberry	600
Cheese	620
Cherry	600
Lemon/Apricot	610
Raspberry Cheese	610
Red Raspberry	600
Bundtlette (4 oz.)	
Banana Chocolate Chip	410
Candied Apple	400
Double Chocolate	440
Sour Cream Coffee Cake	400
Cheesecakes (1 Slice)	
Bailey's®	573
Cappuccino	573
Carrot Layer	500
Funky Chunky	480
Pecan Turtle	609
Snickers®	410
Cookies (1)	
Chocolate Chip Oatmeal	290
Chocolate Chip	410
Oatmeal Raisin	350
Peanut Butter	430
Shortbread	380
Triple Chocolate Chunk	200
White Chocolate Macadamia	420
Dressings	
Thousand Island, 2 oz.	140
Asian Sesame Ginger, 1 oz.	128
Bleu Cheese, 2 oz.	140
Caesar, 2 Tblsp	150
Dill Sauce, .25 oz.	30
Fat-free Ranch, 2 Tblsp	20
Fat-free Raspberry Vinaigrette, 2 Tblsp	25
Fat-free Toasted Sesame, 2 Tblsp	50

Greek, 2 Tblsp	100
House Italian, 2 oz.	100
Vinaigrette, 2 Tblsp	100

Auntie Anne's

Pretzels	Calories
Almond Pretzel	350
Almond Pretzel w/butter	400
Cinnamon Sugar Pretzel	350
Cinnamon Sugar Pretzel w/butter	450
Garlic Pretzel	320
Garlic Pretzel w/butter	350
Glazin' Raisin® Pretzel	470
Glazin' Raisin® Pretzel w/butter	510
Jalapeño Pretzel	270
Jalapeño Pretzel w/butter	310
Kidstix - Cinnamon Sugar	233
Kidstix - Cinnamon Sugar w/butter	300
Kidstix - Original	227
Kidstix - Original w/butter	247
Original Pretzel	340
Original Pretzel w/butter	370
Parmesan Herb Pretzel	390
Parmesan Herb Pretzel w/butter	440
Sesame Pretzel	350
Sesame Pretzel w/butter	410
Sour Cream & Onion Pretzel	310
Sour Cream & Onion Pretzel w/butter	340
Whole Wheat Pretzel	350
Whole Wheat Pretzel w/butter	370
Dipping Sauces	
Light Cream Cheese	70
Strawberry Cream Cheese	110
Caramel Dip	135
Cheese Sauce	100
Chocolate Flavored Dip	130
Marinara Sauce	10
Sweet Mustard	60
Hot Salsa Cheese	100
Dutch Ice®	
Grape Dutch Ice® 14 fl. oz.	180
Grape Dutch Ice® 20 fl. oz.	260
Kiwi-Banana Dutch Ice® 14 fl. oz.	190
Kiwi-Banana Dutch Ice® 20 fl. oz.	270
Lemonade Dutch Ice® 14 fl. oz.	315
Lemonade Dutch Ice® 20 fl. oz.	450
Mocha Dutch Ice® 14 fl. oz.	400
Mocha Dutch Ice® 20 fl. oz.	570
Orange Crème Dutch Ice® 14 fl. oz.	280

AUNTIE ANNE'S - BACKYARD BURGERS

Orange Crème Dutch Ice® 20 fl. oz.	400
Piña Colada Dutch Ice® 14 fl. oz.	250
Piña Colada Dutch Ice® 20 fl. oz.	360
Blue Raspberry Dutch Ice® 14 fl. oz.	175
Blue Raspberry Dutch Ice® 20 fl. oz.	250
Strawberry Dutch Ice® 14 fl. oz.	220
Strawberry Dutch Ice® 20 fl. oz.	315
Wild Cherry Dutch Ice® 14 fl. oz.	230
Wild Cherry Dutch Ice® 20 fl. oz.	330

Backyard Burgers

Classic Burgers	Calories
1/3 Lb. Back Yard Burger	470
1/3 Lb. Back Yard Cheeseburger	520
Great Little Burger	280
Specialty Burgers	
Bacon Cheddar Burger	620
Barbeque Bacon Burger	630
Black Jack Burger	580
Chili Cheese Burger	560
Hawaiian Burger	550
Miz Grazi Burger	530
Mushroom Swiss Burger	540
Worcestershire Burger	530
Back Yard Specialties	
Back Yard BLT	270
Back Yard Chili Cheese Dog	400
Back Yard Chili Dog	340
Back Yard Hot Dog	310
Chicken Tenderloins (3 Piece)	400
Gardenburger	140
Dipping Sauces	
Barbeque	50
Gourmet	150
Gravy	70
Honey Mustard	170
Chicken Sandwiches	
Bacon Swiss Chicken Sandwich	390
Barbeque Chicken Sandwich	280
Blackened Chicken Sandwich	290
Buffalo Ranch Chicken Sandwich	540
Hawaiian Chicken Sandwich	280
Honey Mustard Chicken Sandwich	320
Lemon Butter Chicken Sandwich	260
Savory Chicken Sandwich	230
Baked Potatoes And Fries	
Chili And Cheddar	330
Miz Grazi's Chili Cheese Fries	350
Ranch	410
Salsa	250

BACKYARD BURGERS – BAJA FRESH

Seasoned Fries (Regular)	260
Traditional	190
Waffle Fries (Regular)	240
Garden Fresh Salads	
Blackened Chicken Salad	160
Charbroiled Chicken Salad	140
Garden Fresh Salad	25
Salad Dressings	
fat-free Honey Dijon	60
fat-free Italian	20
fat-free Ranch	60
Honey Mustard	140
Italian	200
Ranch	270
Thousand Island	250
Ice Cream	
Chocolate Milkshake	560
Strawberry Milkshake	560
Vanilla (Scoop)	140
Vanilla Milkshake	540
Cobblers	
Apple	430
Blackberry	420
Cherry	460
Peach	420
Strawberry	410
Beverages	
7 Up	200
Code Red Mountain Dew	220
Dr. Pepper	200
Fruitworks Fruit Punch	220
Lemonade	392
Mountain Dew	220
Mug Root Beer	220
Pepsi	200
Sweet Tea	130
Unsweetened Tea	0

Baja Fresh

Burritos	**Calories**
Baja, Chicken	820
Baja, Steak	920
Bare	650
Bean & Cheese, Chicken	1000
Bean & Cheese, Steak	1100
Bean & Cheese, Vegetarian	870
Dos Manos, Chicken	740
Dos Manos, Steak	790
Enchilada Style Dos Manos Add	890

BAJA FRESH

Enchilada Style to any burrito Add	930
Grilled Vegetarian	770
Mexicano, Chicken	830
Mexicano, Steak	920
Ultimo, Chicken	860
Ultimo, Steak	950
Vegetarian Bare	560

Tacos

Baja Fish	270
Baja Mahi Mahi	260
Grilled Veggies	420
Original Baja Style, Chicken	190
Original Baja Style, Shrimp	190
Original Baja Style, Steak	220
Taco Chilito, Chicken	320
Taco Chilito, Steak	340

Salads

Baja Ensalada, Chicken	310
Baja Ensalada, Fish	360
Baja Ensalada, Steak	460
Mahi Mahi Ensalada	280
Shrimp Ensalada	180
Side Salad	70
Side-By-Side	320
Tostada, Chicken	1140
Tostada, Fish	1010
Tostada, Steak	1230

Specialties

Enchiladas Verano	580
Enchiladas Verdes, Charbroiled Chicken	770
Enchiladas Verdes, Cheese	840
Enchiladas Verdes, Vegetarian	720
Enchiladas, Charbroiled Chicken	780
Enchiladas, Charbroiled Steak	890
Enchiladas, Cheese	850
Fajitas, Chicken w/Corn Tortillas	1200
Fajitas, Chicken w/Flour Tortillas	1360
Fajitas, Steak w/Corn Tortillas	1370
Fajitas, Steak w/Flour Tortillas	1530
Mini Quesa-Dita, Charbroiled Chicken	670
Mini Quesa-Dita, Charbroiled Steak	700
Mini Quesa-Dita, Cheese	620
Mini Tosta-Dita, Charbroiled Chicken	570
Mini Tosta-Dita, Charbroiled Steak	630
Nachos, Charbroiled Chicken	2010
Nachos, Charbroiled Steak	2100
Nachos, Cheese	1880
Quesadilla, Charbroiled Chicken	1260
Quesadilla, Charbroiled Steak	1350
Quesadilla, Cheese	1130

Quesadilla, Vegetarian	1180
Taquitos, Charbroiled Chicken w/ Beans	750
Taquitos, Charbroiled Chicken w/ Rice	710
Taquitos, Charbroiled Steak w/ Beans	820
Taquitos, Charbroiled Steak w/Rice	790

Sides

Beans, Black	360
Beans, Pinto	320
Cebollitas	40
Dressing, fat-free Salsa Verde	15
Dressing, Olive Oil Vinaigrette	230
Dressing, Ranch	220
Guacamole, Large	290
Guacamole, Medium	110
Guacamole, Pronto	550
Guacamole, Small	70
Rice	280
Salsa	50
Salsa, Baja	1100

Baskin Robbins

Hard Scoop Ice Cream (Reg Scoop)	Calories
Chocolate	270
Chocolate Chip	270
Jamoca Almond Fudge	280
Pralines 'n Cream	280
Vanilla	250

Sherbets, Ices, Sorbets (Reg. Scoop)

Daiquiri Ice	130
Peachy Keen Sorbet	110
Rainbow Sherbet	16

Low Fat Ice Cream (Reg Scoop)

Espresso 'n Cream	180

Low Fat Yogurt (Small)

Maui Brownie Madness	250

No Sugar Ice Cream (Reg Scoop)

Peach Crumb Pie	180
Thin Mint	160

Soft Serve Non-fat Yogurt (Small)

Chocolate 5 oz.	190

Truly Free Yogurt (Small)

Café Mocha	140

Shakes (Regular)

Chocolate Ice Cream	750
Vanilla Ice Cream	630

Blast (Regular)

Cappuccino Blast w/whipped Cream	340

Smoothie (Regular)

Very Strawberry w/soft Serve Ice Cream	320

Ben & Jerry's

Ice Cream(1/2 Cup)	Calories
Chocolate Fudge Brownie	260
Brownie Batter	310
Butter Pecan	290
Cherry Garcia®	250
Chocolate Chip Cookie Dough	280
Chocolate For A Change™	270
Chocolate Fudge Brownie	280
Chubby Hubby®	330
Chunky Monkey®	300
Coffee For A Change™	240
Coffee Heath® Bar Crunch	310
Everything But The...™	320
Fudge Central™	300
Half Baked™	280
Karamel Sutra™	290
Makin' Whoopie Pie™	270
Mint Chocolate Cookie	270
New York Super Fudge Chunk®	310
Oatmeal Cookie Chunk	280
One Sweet Whirled™	280
Peanut Butter Cup™	380
Peanut Butter Me Up™	330
Phish Food®	280
Pistachio Pistachio™	280
Strawberry	200
Sweet Cream & Cookies	240
Uncanny Cashew™	290
Vanilla	220
Vanilla For A Change™	240
Vanilla Heath® Bar Crunch	300
Frozen Yogurt	
Cherry Garcia®	170
Chocolate Fudge Brownie	190
Half Baked™	210
Phish Food®	230
Peace Pops	
Cherry Garcia	280
Cookie Dough	380
One Sweet Whirled	270
Vanilla	300
Vanilla w/ Heath Toffee	320
Single Containers	
Cherry Garcia	220
Chocolate Fudge Brownie	230
Cookie Dough	240
Vanilla For A Change	200

Blimpie

Cold Subs (6" Reg)	Calories
Blimpie Best	476
Club	440
Ham & Cheese	436
Roast Beef	468
Seafood	355
Tuna	493
Turkey	424
Grilled Subs (6" Reg)	
Beef, Turkey & Cheddar	600
Cuban	462
Pastrami Special	462
Reuben	630
Ultimate Club	724
Hot Subs (6" Reg)	
BLT	588
Buffalo Chicken	400
ChikMax	511
Grilled Chicken	373
Meatball	572
MexiMax	425
Pastrami	507
Steak & Onion Melt	440
VegiMax	395
Breads (6" Reg Unless Noted)	
Flour Tortilla (1 Wrap)	323
Garden Italian	268
Honey Oat	298
Marbled Rye	297
Mediterranean Flat Bread (1)	270
Spinach Tortilla (1 Wrap)	308
Wheat	233
Wheat w/Poppy Seed	240
Wheat w/Sesame Seed	247
White	238
White w/Poppy Seed	245
White w/Sesame Seed	252
Zesty Parmesan	267
Wraps (Reg Size)	
Beef & Cheddar	714
Chicken Caesar	646
Southwestern	674
Steak & Onion	716
Ultimate BLT	831
Zesty Italian	638
Salads (Reg Size)	
Antipasto	244
Chef	212

Chili Ole	480
Grilled Chicken w/Caesar Dressing	347
Roast Beef 'n Blue	390
Seafood	122
Tuna	261
Zesto Pesto Turkey	370

Toppings, Sauces, & Dressings

Caesar (1.5 oz)	208
Cheddar Cheese (1 Slice)	52
Cracked Peppercorn (1.5 oz)	237
Frank's Red Hot Buffalo Sauce (1.0 oz)	13
French's Honey Mustard (1 Tblsp)	5
GourMayo Chipotle Chili (1 Tblsp)	50
GourMayo Sun Dried Tomato (1 Tblsp)	50
GourMayo Wasabi Horseradish (1 Tblsp)	50
Guacamole (1.5 oz)	194
Oil & Vinegar Topping (For 6" sub)	36
Pesto Dressing (1.0 oz)	132
Provolone Or Swiss Cheese (1 Slice)	80

Soups (8 oz)

Chicken w/White & Wild Rice	230
Cream of Broccoli & Cheese	190
Cream of Potato	190
Garden Vegetable	80
Grande Chili w/Beans & Beef	250
Homestyle Chicken Noodle	120
Tomato Basil w/Raviolini	110
Vegetable Beef	80

Sides (5 oz Or 1 Bag)

Cole Slaw	180
Macaroni Salad	360
Mustard Potato Salad	160
Potato Salad	270
Potato Chips Any Flavor	210

Cookies (1 Cookie)

Chocolate Chunk	200
Macadamia White Chunk	210
Oatmeal Raisin	190
Peanut Butter	220
Sugar	330

59

EATING OUT

Bojangles

Cajun Spiced Chicken	Calories
Breast	278
Leg	264
Thigh	310
Wing	355
Southern Style Chicken	
Breast	261
Leg	254

Thigh	308
Wing	337
Sweet Biscuits	
Bo Berry™	220
Cinnamon	320
Biscuit Sandwiches	
Biscuit (plain)	243
Bacon	290
Bacon, Egg & Cheese	550
Cajun Filet	454
Country Ham	270
Egg	400
Sausage	350
Smoked Sausage	380
Steak	649
Sandwiches	
Cajun Filet (without mayo)	337
Cajun Filet (w/mayo)	437
Grilled Filet (without mayo)	235
Grilled Filet (w/mayo)	335
Individual Fixin'	
Botato Rounds	235
Cajun Pintos	110
Marinated Cole Slaw	136
Corn On The Cob	140
Dirty Rice	166
Green Beans	25
Macaroni & Cheese	198
Potatoes w/o Gravy	80
Seasoned Fries	344
Snacks	
Chicken Supremes	337
Buffalo Bites	180

Boston Market

Entrees	Calories
Dark Meat Chicken, No Skin	190
Dark Meat Chicken, w/Skin	320
White Meat Chicken, No Skin or Wing	170
White Meat Chicken, w/Skin Or Wing	280
Chicken w/Skin	590
Chicken Pot Pie	750
Chunky Chicken Salad	480
Grilled Chicken BBQ	400
Grilled Chicken Teriyaki	290
Honey Glazed Ham (Lean)	210
Marinated Grilled Chicken	230
Meat Loaf	310
Meat Loaf & Brown Gravy	360

BOSTON MARKET

Meat Loaf & Chunky Tomato Sauce	350
Skinless Chicken Rotisserie Turkey Breast	170
Turkey Pot Pie	710

Sandwiches (1 Sandwich)

BBQ Grilled Chicken	830
BBQ Grilled Chicken (no mayo or cheese)	550
Chicken (no cheese or sauce)	400
Chicken (w/cheese and sauce)	640
Ham (no cheese or sauce	420
Ham (w/cheese and sauce)	660
Marinated Grilled Chicken	670
Marinated Grilled Chicken (no mayo)	470
Meat Loaf w/Cheese	730
Open Faced Meatloaf w/Potatoes & Gravy	730
Open Faced Turkey	720
Shredded BBQ Chicken	590
Teriyaki Grilled Chicken	650
Turkey Bacon Club	770
Turkey (no cheese or sauce	400
Turkey (w/cheese & sauce)	630

Sides (1 Serving)

Butternut Squash	150
Caesar Side Salad	300
Chicken Gravy	15
Chunky Chicken Salad	480
Cole Slaw	300
Cranberry Walnut Relish	350
Creamed Spinach	260
Fruit Salad	70
Green Bean Casserole	80
Green Beans	70
Homestyle Mashed Potatoes	210
Homestyle Mashed Potatoes w/Gravy	230
Hot Cinnamon Apples	250
Jumping Juice Squares	150
New Potatoes	130
Old fashioned Potato Salad	200
Rice Pilaf	140
Savory Stuffing	190
Steamed Vegetables	30
Sweet Potato Casserole	280
Tortellini Salad	350
Whole Kernel Corn	180

Soup (3/4 Cup)

Chicken Noodle	100
Chicken Tortilla No Toppings	80
Chicken Tortilla w/Toppings	170
Turkey Tortilla No Toppings	70
Turkey Tortilla w/Toppings	160

Salads

Caesar Entrée	470
Grilled Chicken Caesar	710
Oriental Grill Chicken No Dressing & Chips	320
Oriental Grill Chicken w/Dressing & Chips	660
Southwest Grill Chicken No Dressing & Chips	470
Southwest Grill Chicken w/Dressing & Chips	890

Baked Goods (1 Cookie Or Slice)

Apple Streusel Pie	460
Brownie	580
Cheesecake	600
Cherry Streusel Pie	360
Chocolate Cake	650
Chocolate Chip Cookie	390
Cornbread	200
Family Brownie	160
Hummingbird Cake	710
Oatmeal Scotchie Cookie	390
Oreo Brownie w/Chocolate Chips	840
Peanut Butter Chip Cookie	420
Pecan Pie	500
Pumpkin Pie	290
Rice Krispie Treat	420

Breugger's Bagels

Bagels	**Calories**
Blueberry	330
Chocolate chip	310
Cinnamon Raisin	320
Cinnamon Sugar	340
Cranberry Orange	330
Everything	310
Garlic	310
Honey Grain	330
Jalapeno	310
Onion	310
Plain	300
Poppy	310
Pumpernickel	320
Rosemary Olive Oil	350
Salt	300
Sesame	320
Sun Dried Tomato	320

Breakfast Sandwiches (On Plain Bagel)

Egg & Cheese	480
Egg, Cheese, & Bacon	560
Egg, Cheese, & Ham	520
Egg, Cheese, & Sausage	680

BREUGGER'S BAGELS – BRUSTER'S

Cream Cheese Spreads (2 Tblsp)

Bacon Scallion	100
Chive	100
Garden Veggie	0
Garden Veggie Light	60
Herb & Garlic Light	70
Honey Walnut	110
Jalapeno	100
Olive Pimento	100
Plain	90
Plain Light	70
Smoked Salmon	100
Strawberry Light	70
Wildberry	100

Deli Sandwiches (On Plain Bagel)

Chicken Breast	440
Chicken Salad w/mayo	460
Ham w/honey mustard	440
Hummus 2 Tblsp (add bagel)	60
Tuna Salad (add bagel)	180
Turkey w/Mayo	480

Bagel Sandwiches (on plain bagel)

Atlantic Smoked Salmon	470
Chicken Fajita	500
Garden Veggie	390
Herby Turkey	530
Leonardo Da Veggie	460
Santa Fe Turkey	480

Desserts

Blondie Bar	370
Breugger's Bars	420
Cappuccino Bars	420
Chocolate Chunk Brownie	330
Luscious Lemon Bar	350
Mint Brownie	300
Oatmeal Cranberry Mountains	430
Pecan Chocolate Chunk Bar	350
Raspberry Sammies	270

Bruster's

No Sugar Added-Fat Free Ice Cream (1/2 Cup)	Calories
Chocolate	100
Chocolate Caramel Swirl	120
Chocolate Fudge Ripple	120
Chocolate Raspberry Swirl	110
Cinnamon	100
Vanilla	100
Vanilla Caramel Swirl	110
Vanilla Fudge Ripple	110
Vanilla Raspberry Swirl	110

Burger King

Breakfast	Calories
Croissant w/Egg, & Cheese	320
Croissant w/Sausage & Cheese	420
Croissant w/Sausage, Egg, & Cheese	520
French Toast Sticks (5 sticks)	390
Hash Brown Rounds, Large	390
Hash Brown Rounds, Small	230
Sourdough w/Bacon, Egg, & Cheese	380
Sourdough w/Ham, Egg, & Cheese	380
Sourdough w/Sausage, Egg, & Cheese	540
Burgers & Sandwiches	
Bacon Cheeseburger	400
Bacon Double Cheeseburger	580
Cheeseburger	360
Chicken Specialty	560
Chicken Specialty (no mayo)	460
Chicken Tenders 4 Pieces	170
Chicken Tenders 5 Pieces	210
Chicken Tenders 6 Pieces	250
Chicken Tenders 8 Pieces	340
Chicken Whopper	580
Chicken Whopper (no mayo)	420
Chicken Whopper Jr.	350
Chicken Whopper Jr. (no mayo)	270
Double Cheeseburger	540
Double Hamburger	450
Double Whopper	980
Double Whopper (no mayo)	820
Double Whopper w/cheese	1070
Double Whopper w/cheese (no mayo)	910
Fish Filet	520
Hamburger	310
King Supreme	550
Veggie Burger	330
Veggie Burger w/reduced fat mayo	290
Veggie Burger w/Regular Mayo	390
Whopper	710
Whopper (no mayo)	550
Whopper w/Cheese	800
Whopper w/Cheese (no mayo)	640
Whopper Jr.	390
Whopper Jr. (no mayo)	310
Whopper Jr. w/cheese	440
Whopper Jr. w/cheese (no mayo)	360
Sides	
Baked Potato w/chives	260
Chili	190
French Fries, King	600

BURGER KING – CAPTAIN D'S

French Fries, Large	500
French Fries, Medium	360
French Fries, Small	230
French Fries, Value	340
Onion Rings, King	550
Onion Rings, Large	480
Onion Rings, Medium	320
Onion Rings, Small	180
Onion Rings, Value	280
Salads	
Chicken Caesar (no dressing or croutons)	160
Side Garden (no dressing)	25
Desserts, Shakes, & Drinks	
Chocolate Chip Cookie	440
Dutch Apple Pie	340
Frozen, Cherry - Large	450
Frozen, Cherry - Medium	370
Frozen, Cola - Large	460
Frozen, Cola - Medium	370
Orange Juice	140
Shake, Chocolate - Medium	790
Shake, Chocolate - Small	620
Shake, Strawberry - Medium	780
Shake, Strawberry - Small	620
Shake, Vanilla - Medium	720
Shake, Vanilla - Small	560
Shake, Vanilla - Value	410
Sunday Pie	300

Captain D's

Item	Calories
Broiled Chicken Breast	102
Broiled Chicken Lunch	503
Broiled Chicken Platter	802
Broiled Fish & Chicken Lunch	478
Broiled Fish & Chicken Platter	777
Broiled Fish Lunch	435
Broiled Fish Platter	734
Broiled Shrimp Lunch	421
Broiled Shrimp Platter	720
Fried Chicken Salad	498
Gumbo	172
Stuffed Crab	91
Sandwich	
Broiled Chicken	451
Broiled Fish	530
Giant Fish Sandwich	649
Side Items	
Baked Potato	278

Breadstick	113
Cheese sticks	218
Cob Corn	251
Cocktail Sauce	137
Cole Slaw	158
Crackers	50
Cracklins	218
French Fried Potatoes	302
Fried Okra	300
Green Beans (Seasoned)	46
Hushpuppies	756
Hushpuppy (1)	126
Rice	124
Salad	20
Slice of Cheese	54
Vegetable Medley	36
White Beans	126
Dressings and Sauces	
Blue Cheese	105
French	111
Honey Mustard	160
Ranch	92
Light Italian Dressing	16
Sweet & Sour Sauce	52
Tartar Sauce	75
Margarine	102
Imitation Sour Cream	29
Desserts	
Carrot Cake	434
Cheesecake	420
Chocolate Cake	303
Pecan Pie	458
Pineapple Cream Cheese Pie	340

66

EATING OUT

Caribou

Hot and Cold Drinks	Calories
2% Cappuccino, 12 oz.	122
2% Cappuccino, 16 oz.	162
2% Cappuccino, 20 oz.	203
2% Chai Latte, 12 oz.	215
2% Chai Latte, 16 oz.	286
2% Chai Latte, 20 oz.	358
2% Latte, 12 oz.	129
2% Latte, 16 oz.	171
2% Latte, 20 oz.	214
2% Mocha, 12 oz.	260
2% Mocha, 16 oz.	347
2% Mocha, 20 oz.	434
Caramel Cooler, 12 oz.	362

CARIBOU

Caramel Cooler, 16 oz.	450
Caramel Cooler, 20 oz.	538
Caramel Hirise, 16 oz.	266
Caramel Hirise, 20 oz.	332
Chocolate Cooler, 12 oz.	193
Chocolate Cooler, 16 oz.	257
Chocolate Cooler, 20 oz.	321
Coffee Cooler, 12 oz.	173
Coffee Cooler, 16 oz.	230
Coffee Cooler, 20 oz.	288
Espresso Cooler, 12 oz.	136
Espresso Cooler, 16 oz.	193
Espresso Cooler, 20 oz.	251
Hot Apple Blast, 12 oz.	305
Hot Apple Blast, 16 oz.	379
Hot Apple Blast, 20 oz.	452
Lite White Berry, 16 oz.	311
Lite White Berry, 20 oz.	389
Mint Condition, 16 oz.	374
Mint Condition, 20 oz.	468
Mint Oreo Cooler, 12 oz.	494
Mint Oreo Cooler, 16 oz.	614
Mint Oreo Cooler, 20 oz.	735
Raspberry Smoothie, 12 oz.	220
Raspberry Smoothie, 16 oz.	293
Raspberry Smoothie, 20 oz.	367
Skim Cappuccino, 12 oz.	84
Skim Cappuccino, 16 oz.	113
Skim Cappuccino, 20 oz.	141
Skim Chai, 12 oz.	177
Skim Chai, 16 oz.	236
Skim Chai, 20 oz.	295
Skim Latte, 12 oz.	91
Skim Latte, 16 oz.	121
Skim Latte, 20 oz.	152
Skim Mocha, 12 oz.	226
Skim Mocha, 16 oz.	302
Skim Mocha, 20 oz.	378
Straw Ban Smoothie, 12 oz.	190
Straw Ban Smoothie, 16 oz.	253
Straw Ban Smoothie, 20 oz.	316
Turtle Mocha, 16 oz.	374
Turtle Mocha, 20 oz.	468
Vanilla Cooler, 12 oz.	193
Vanilla Cooler, 16 oz.	257
Vanilla Cooler, 20 oz.	321
Wild Berry Smoothie, 12 oz.	176
Wild Berry Smoothie, 16 oz.	235
Wild Berry Smoothie, 20 oz.	293

Chick-Fil-A

Breakfast Items	Calories
Bacon Platter	525
Biscuit, plain	260
Biscuit and gravy	310
Biscuit w/bacon	300
Biscuit w/bacon & egg	390
Biscuit w/bacon, cheese, & egg	430
Biscuit w/egg	340
Biscuit w/egg & cheese	390
Biscuit w/sausage	410
Biscuit w/sausage & egg	500
Biscuit w/sausage, cheese, & egg	540
Chicken Biscuit	400
Chicken Biscuit w/cheese	450
Chicken Platter	589
Danish	430
Hashbrowns	170
Sausage Platter	603
Sandwiches & Specialties	
CharGrilled Chicken Club Sandwich	360
CharGrilled Chicken Deluxe Sandwich	280
CharGrilled Chicken Filet No Bun Or Pickle	100
CharGrilled Chicken Sandwich	280
CharGrilled Chicken Sandwich No Butter	240
Chicken Deluxe Sandwich	420
Chicken Filet No Bun Or Pickle	230
Chicken Salad Sandwich (On Whole Wheat)	350
Chicken Sandwich	410
Chicken Sandwich No Butter	380
Chicken Soup (1 Cup)	100
Chick-N-Strips (4 Count)	250
Cool Wrap, CharGrilled Chicken	390
Cool Wrap, Chicken Caesar	460
Cool Wrap, Spicy Chicken	390
Nuggets (8 pack)	260
Salads	
CharGrilled Chicken Garden	180
CharGrilled Chicken Caesar	240
Chick-N-Strips	340
Side Salad	80
Sides & Sauces (1 Pack)	
Carrot & Raisin Salad, Small	130
Cole Slaw, Small	210
Croutons, Garlic & Butter	90
Fries, Small	280
Sauce, Barbeque	45
Sauce, Dijon Honey Mustard	50

Sauce, Honey Mustard	45
Sauce, Polynesian	110
Sunflower Kernels, Roasted	80

Dressings (1 Pack)

Basil Vinaigrette	210
Blue Cheese	190
Buttermilk Ranch	190
Caesar	200
fat-free Dijon Honey Mustard	60
Light Italian	20
Spicy	210
Thousand Island	170

Dessert

Cheescake slice	340
Cheesecake slice w/blueberry topping	370
Cheesecake slice w/strawberry topping	360
Fudge Nut Brownie	330
Icedream, small cone	160
Icedream, small cup	230
Lemon Pie slice	320

Drinks

Diet Lemonade, Small	25
Iced Tea Sweet, Small	80
Lemonade, Small	170

Chuck E. Cheese

Appetizers	**Calories**
Bread Sticks (1)	370
Buffalo Wings (4 Pieces)	220
French Fries (7 Pieces)	283
Mozzarella Sticks (2 sticks)	380
Pizza Sauce (1/4 Cup)	35

Sandwiches

Grilled Chicken Sub	740
Ham & Cheese	770
Hot Dog	430
Italian Sub	770

Pizza (2 Medium Slices)

BBQ Chicken	410
Beef	411
Cheese	330
Pepperoni	371
Sausage	387

Salad Bar/Dressings (2 Tblsp)

Blue Cheese	170
Catalina	35
Lite Ranch	80
Olive Oil & Vinegar	90
Thousand Island	110

CHUCK E. CHEESE – CINNABON

Cake (1/12 cake)

8" Chocolate Cake w/whipped cream	208
8" White Cake w/whipped cream	208

Church's

Main Items	Calories
Breast, fried	200
Breast, no batter or skin	145
Krispy Tender Strips (1 piece)	137
Leg, fried	140
Leg, no batter or skin	118
Tender Crunchers (6-8 pieces)	411
Thigh, fried	230
Thigh, no batter or skin	180
Wing, fried	250
Wing, no batter or skin	160

Sides	
Cajun Rice, Reg	130
Cole Slaw, Reg	92
Collard Greens, Reg	25
Corn on the Cob (1 piece)	139
French Fries, Reg	210
Fried Steak w/white gravy (1 piece)	470
Honey Butter Biscuit (1)	250
Jalapeno Cheese Bombers (4)	240
Macaroni & Cheese, Reg	210
Mashed Potatoes & gravy – regular	90
Okra – regular	210
Sweet Corn Nuggets, Reg	250
Whole Jalapeno Peppers (2)	10

Sauces (1 Package)	
BBQ	29
Creamy Jalapeno	102
Honey Mustard	111
Purple Pepper	46
Sweet & Sour	31

Dessert (1 pie)	
Apple Pie	280
Double Lemon Pie	300
Strawberry Cream Cheese Pie	280

Cinnabon

Item	Calories
Caramel Pecanbon (1 roll)	1100
Cinnabon (1 roll)	730
Cinnabon Stix (5-count)	350
Cinnapack 6-pack To-Go Box (1/2 roll)	440
Minibon (1 roll)	300
Mochalatte Chill	410

COLDSTONE CREAMERY – DAIRY QUEEN

ColdStone Creamery

Item (4 oz.)	Calories
Chocolate Ice Cream	245
Italian Sorbet	110
Sweet Cream Ice Cream	255
Yogurt	135

Dairy Queen

Cones	Calories
Chocolate Cone – large	340
Chocolate Cone – medium	340
Chocolate Cone – small	240
Chocolate Soft Serve, 1/2 cup	150
Dipped Cone – small	490
Vanilla Cone – large	410
Vanilla Cone – medium	330
Vanilla Cone, Small	230
Vanilla Soft Serve, 1/2 Cup	140
Malts, Shakes, Slushes	
Chocolate Malt, Small	650
Chocolate Malt, Medium	880
Chocolate Shake, Small	560
Chocolate Shake, Medium	770
Frozen Hot Chocolate	860
Misty Slush, Small	220
Misty Slush, Medium	290
Sundaes & Royal Treats	
Banana Split	510
Brownie Earthquake	740
Chocolate Sundae, Medium	400
Chocolate Sundae, Small	280
Peanut Buster Parfait	730
Pecan Mudslide Treat	650
Strawberry Shortcake	430
Novelties	
Buster Bar	450
Chocolate Dilly Bar	210
DQ Sandwich	200
Fudge Bar – No Sugar Added	50
Lemon Freez'r	80
Starkiss	80
Vanilla Orange Bar - No Sugar Added	60
Blizzards	
Chocolate Chip Cookie Dough, Medium	950
Chocolate Chip Cookie Dough, Small	660
Chocolate Sandwich Cookie, Medium	640
Chocolate Sandwich Cookie, Small	520

Treatzza Pizza and Cake (1/8 of Whole)

Frozen 8" Round Cake	370
Heath Pizza	180
Layered 8" Round Cake	330
M&Ms Pizza	190

Sandwich and Sides

Bacon Double Cheeseburger	610
BBQ Beef Sandwich	300
BBQ Pork Sandwich	280
Cheeseburger	340
Chicken Breast Filet Sandwich	500
Chicken Strip Basket	1000
Chili'n'Cheese Dog	330
Crispy Chicken Salad, Fat-free Italian	460
Crispy Chicken Salad, Honey Mustard	700
Double Cheeseburger	540
French Fries, Medium	440
French Fries, Small	350
Grilled Chicken Salad, Fat-free Italian	230
Grilled Chicken Salad, Honey Mustard	470
Grilled Chicken Sandwich	310
Hamburger	290
Hot Dog	240
Onion Rings	320
Super Dog	580
Super Dog w/Chili'n'Cheese	710
Ultimate Burger	670

Del Taco

Combo Meal w/Drink	**Calories**
#1 Combo Burrito, Fries	1020
#2 Del Classic Chicken Burrito, Fries	1050
#3 Spicy Chicken Burrito, Fries	970
#4 Two Chicken Soft Tacos, Fries	910
#5 Ultimate Taco, Chicken Cheddar Quesadilla	980
#6 Two Tacos, Quesadilla	960
#7 Macho Combo Burrito, Fries	1540
#8 Two Big Fat Steak Tacos, Fries	1270
#8 Two Big Fat Chicken Tacos, Fries	1170
#9 Double Del Cheeseburger, Fries	1050

Tacos

Big Fat Chicken Taco™	340
Big Fat Steak Taco™	390
Big Fat Taco™	320
Chicken Soft Taco	210
Soft Taco	160
Taco	160
Ultimate Taco	260

DEL TACO

Burritos

Bean & Cheese Green Burrito	280
Bean & Cheese Red Burrito	270
Chicken Works Burrito	520
Del Beef Burrito™	550
Del Classic Chicken Burrito™	560
Del Combo Burrito	530
Deluxe Combo Burrito™	570
Deluxe Del Beef Burrito ™	590
Half Pound Green Burrito	430
Half Pound Red Burrito	430
Macho Beef Burrito™	1170
Macho Chicken Burrito™	930
Macho Combo Burrito™	1050
Spicy Chicken Burrito	480
Steak Works Burrito	590
Veggie Works Burrito	490

Quesadillas

Cheddar Quesadilla	500
Chicken Cheddar Quesadilla	580
Spicy Jack Chicken Quesadilla	570
Spicy Jack Quesadilla	490

Salads

Deluxe Chicken Salad	740
Deluxe Taco Salad™	780
Taco Salad	350

Burgers

Bacon Double Del Cheeseburger™	610
Bun Taco	440
Cheeseburger	330
Del Cheeseburger™	430
Double Del Cheeseburger™	560
Hamburger	280

Nachos

Macho Nachos	1100
Nachos	380

Sides

Beans 'n Cheese Cup	260
Rice Cup	140

Fries

Chili Cheese Fries	670
Deluxe Chili Cheese Fries™	710
Large Fries	490
Macho Fries	690
Regular Fries	350
Small Fries	210

Breakfast

Bacon & Egg Quesadilla	450
Breakfast Burrito	250
Egg & Cheese Burrito	450

DEL TACO – DENNY'S

Macho Bacon & Egg Burrito™	1030
Steak & Egg Burrito	580
Side of Bacon (2 slices)	50
Shakes	
Large Chocolate Shake	680
Large Strawberry Shake	540
Large Vanilla Shake	550
Small Chocolate Shake	520
Small Strawberry Shake	410
Small Vanilla Shake	420
Drinks	
Coffee	0
Macho Iced Tea	10
Milk – 1% low-fat	130
Orange Juice	140

Denny's

Breakfast	Calories
Bacon, 4 Strips	162
Bagel, Dry	235
Belgian Waffle	304
Breakfast Dagwood	1251
Buttermilk Hotcakes	491
Country Fried Potatoes	394
Country Fried Steak & Eggs	430
Egg Beaters® Egg Substitute	71
Egg, One	120
Egg, Two Breakfast	825
English Muffin – dry	125
French Toast	939
Grits	80
Ham, Grilled Slice	94
Hashed Browns Covered	318
Hashed Browns Covered & Smothered	359
Hashed Browns – Plain	218
Moons Over My Hammy	922
Oatmeal'n'Fixins	460
Omelette, Ham'n'Cheddar	581
Omelette, Ultimate	564
Omelette, Veggie-Cheese	480
Sausage, 4 Links	354
Sirloin Steak & Eggs	622
Skillet, Big Texas Chicken Fajita	1217
Skillet, Meat Lover's	1147
Slam, All American	712
Slam, Farmer's	1200
Slam, French	1133
Slam, Lumberjack	1128
Slam, Original Grand	795
Slam, Shamrock	866

DENNY'S

Slam, Slim (no topping)	438
Slugger, Grand Slam	789
T-Bone Steak & Eggs	991
Toast, Dry	90
Topping, blueberry	106
Topping, cherry	86
Topping, strawberry	115

Appetizers

Buffalo Chicken Strips (5)	734
Buffalo Wings (12)	856
Chicken Strips (5)	720
Mozzarella Sticks (8)	710
Sampler	1405
Smothered Cheese Fries	767

Sides

AppleSauce	60
Baked Potato, plain w/skin	220
Bread Stuffing, plain	100
Carrots in Honey Glaze	80
Corn in Butter Sauce	120
Cottage Cheese	72
French Fries	423
Green Beans w/bacon	60
Green peas w/butter sauce	100
Mashed Potatoes, plain	105
Onion Rings	381
Seasoned Fries	261
Sliced Tomatoes (3)	13
Vegetable Rice Pilaf	85

Entrees

Chicken Strips	635
Country Fried Steak	265
Fried Shrimp & Shrimp Scampi	346
Fried Shrimp Dinner	219
Grilled Chicken Breast Dinner	130
Pot Roast Dinner, w/gravy	292
Roast Turkey & Stuffing w/gravy	388
Shrimp Scampi Skillet Dinner	289
Sirloin Steak Dinner	337
Steak & Shrimp Dinner	645
T-Bone Steak Dinner	860

Salads

Deluxe Caesar w/Grilled Chicken Breast, w/dressing	600
Garden Deluxe w/Buffalo Chicken Strips	516
Garden Deluxe w/Chicken Breast	264
Garden Deluxe w/Fried Chicken Strips	438
Garden Deluxe w/Tuna Salad	444
Garden Deluxe w/Turkey & Ham	322
Side Caesar w/dressing	362
Side Garden, no dressing	113

DENNY'S

Sandwiches

BBQ Chicken	1072
BLT	610
Buffalo Chicken	803
Burger, Bacon-Cheddar	875
Burger, Big Texas BBQ	929
Burger, Boca	616
Burger, Classic	673
Burger, Classic w/cheese	836
Burger, Double Decker	1377
Burger, Garlic Mushroom Swiss	872
Club	718
Grilled Chicken	520
Ham & Swiss on Rye	533
Patty Melt	788
Tuna Melt – Albacore	640
Rueben	586
Super Bird	620
Turkey Breast w/Multigrain	476

Soup

Chicken Noodle	60
Clam Chowder	624
Cream of Broccoli	574
Vegetable Beef	79

Desserts

Apple Pie	470
Banana Split	894
Cheesecake	590
Cheesecake Pie (no topping)	470
Chocolate Chunks & Chips Pie	600
Chocolate Layer Cake	275
Chocolate Peanut Butter Pie	653
Cookies & Creme Pie	651
Double Scoop, Sundae	375
Floats	280
Grasshopper Blender Blaster	735
Grasshopper Sundae	734
Hot Fudge Cake Sundae	620
Malted Milkshake	583
Milkshake	560
Single Scoop Sundae	188

Sauces, Dressings and Condiments

BBQ Sauce	47
Brown Gravy	13
Chicken Gravy	14
Country Gravy	17
Dressing, Blue Cheese	163
Dressing, Caesar	133
Dressing, fat-free Ranch	25
Dressing, French	106

DENNY'S – DOMINO'S PIZZA

Dressing, Honey Mustard	160
Dressing, Low Calorie Italian	15
Dressing, Ranch	129
Dressing, Thousand Island	118
Marinara Sauce	48
Sour Cream	91
Tarter Sauce	230

Dippin Dots

Item (5 oz.)	Calories
Flavored Ice	50
Flavored Sherbet	100
Ice Cream	190
No Sugar Added, No-Fat Fudge	60
No Sugar Added, Reduced Fat Vanilla Ice Cream	120
Non-Fat Yogurt	110

Domino's Pizza

12" Specialty Pizza (1 Slice)	Calories
Hand Tossed America's Favorite Feast	255
Hand Tossed Bacon Cheeseburger Feast	275
Hand Tossed Barbeque Feast	255
Hand Tossed Deluxe Feast	230
Hand Tossed ExtravaganZZa Feast	285
Hand Tossed Hawaiian Feast	225
Hand Tossed MeatZZa Feast	300
Hand Tossed Pepperoni Feast	270
Hand Tossed Veggie Feast	220
14" Specialty Pizza (1 Slice)	
Hand Tossed America's Favorite Feast	350
Hand Tossed Bacon Cheeseburger Feast	380
Hand Tossed Barbeque Feast	345
Hand Tossed Deluxe Feast	315
Hand Tossed ExtravaganZZa Feast	385
Hand Tossed Hawaiian Feast	310
Hand Tossed MeatZZa Feast	375
Hand Tossed Pepperoni Feast	365
Hand Tossed Veggie Feast	300
12" Cheese Pizza (1 Slice)	
Deep Dish	240
Hand Tossed	190
Thin Crust (1/4 Pizza)	275
12" Pizza Toppings (Calories Per Slice)	
Anchovies	15
Bacon	50
Beef	40
Cheddar Cheese	30
Extra Cheese	25
Green Olives	10

Ham	10
Italian Sausage	40
Pepperoni	40
Pineapple	6
Ripe Olives	10
14" Cheese Pizza (1 Slice)	
Deep Dish	340
Hand Tossed	260
Thin Crust (1/4 Pizza)	380
14" Pizza Toppings (Calories Per Slice)	
Anchovies	20
Bacon	75
Beef	55
Cheddar Cheese	35
Extra Cheese	35
Green Olives	15
Ham	15
Italian Sausage	55
Pepperoni	50
Pineapple	10
Ripe Olives	15
Sides	
Blue Cheese (1.5 oz Cup)	225
Bread Sticks (1)	115
Buffalo Chicken Kickers (1)	50
Cheesy Bread (1)	140
Cinna Stix (1 Serving)	110
Domino Dots (1 Servnig)	100
Ranch Dressing (1.5 oz Cup)	200
Sweet Icing (2.5 oz Cup)	400
Wings, Barbeque (1)	50
Wings, Hot (1)	45

Donato's Pizza

Pizza, Original Crust	Calories
Serving: 7" Individual Pizza Or 1/4 of A 14" Pizza	
Chicken Veggie Medley	500
Founders	737
Hawaiian	620
Mariachi Beef	613
Mariachi Chicken	580
Original	660
Serious Cheese	640
Serious Meat	817
Veggie	564
Works	729
Pizza, Traditional Crust	
Serving: 7" Individual Pizza Or 1/4 of A 14" Pizza	
Chicken Veggie Medley	647
Founders	900

DONATO'S PIZZA – DUNKIN DONUTS

Hawaiian	794
Mariachi Beef	797
Mariachi Chicken	770
Original	928
Serious Cheese	830
Serious Meat	977
Veggie	752
Works	892
Subs, Whole Sub	
Big Don, Italian	705
Big Don, Lite Italian	631
Grilled Chicken	786
Ham & Cheese, Italian	609
Ham & Cheese, Lite Italian	534
Southwest Turkey	710
Steak & Cheese	929
Veggie, Italian	730
Veggie, Lite Italian	661
Salads	
Grilled Chicken	314
Italian Chef	338
Side	106
Dressings (1.5 oz)	
Italian	230
Lite Italian	20
Sides	
Breadsticks (2)	220
Three Cheese Garlic Bread (whole bun)	605
Dessert Pizza, 1/4 of 14" Pizza	
Apple	722
Cherry	818

Dunkin DoNuts

Beverages (10 oz Unless Noted)	Calories
Coffee	5
Coffee Coolatta w/ 2% milk (16 oz)	240
Coffee Coolatta w/ cream (16 oz)	370
Coffee Coolatta w/ milk (16 oz)	260
Coffee Coolatta w/ skim milk (16 oz)	230
Coffee w/cream	60
Coffee w/cream & sugar	90
Coffee w/milk	25
Coffee w/milk & sugar	70
Coffee w/skim milk	15
Coffee w/skim milk & sugar	60
Coffee w/sugar	50
Dunkaccino	250
Hot Chocolate	210
Iced Coffee (16 oz)	5

DUNKIN DONUTS

Iced Coffee w/cream (16 oz)	60
Iced Coffee w/cream & sugar (16 oz)	110
Iced Coffee w/milk (16 oz)	25
Iced Coffee w/milk & sugar (16 oz)	70
Iced Coffee w/skim milk (16 oz)	20
Iced Coffee w/skim milk & sugar (16 oz)	60
Iced Coffee w/sugar (16 oz)	50
Fruit Coolatta, Orange Mango (16 oz)	280
Fruit Coolatta, Strawberry (16 oz)	270
Vanilla Bean Coolatta (16 oz)	440
Vanilla Chai	220

DoNuts

Apple Crumb	230
Apple Fritter	300
Apple N' Spice	200
Bavarian Kreme	210
Bismarck, Chocolate Iced	340
Black Raspberry	210
Blueberry Cake	290
Blueberry Crumb	240
Boston Kreme	240
Bow Tie	300
Butternut Cake Ring	300
Chocolate Coconut Cake	300
Chocolate Frosted Cake	300
Chocolate Frosted Coffee Roll	290
Chocolate Frosted	200
Chocolate Glazed Cake	290
Chocolate Kreme Filled	270
Cinnamon Bun	510
Cinnamon Cake	270
Coconut Cake	290
Coffee Roll	270
Double Chocolate Cake	310
Dunkin' Donut	240
Éclair	270
Glazed Cake	270
Glazed Chocolate Fritter	280
Glazed Crullers	290
Glazed	180
Glazed Fritter	260
Jelly Filled	210
Jelly Stick	290
Lemon	200
Maple Frosted Coffee Roll	290
Maple Frosted	210
Marble Frosted	200
Old Fashioned Cake	250
Plain Cruller	240
Powdered Cake	270

DUNKIN DONUTS

Powdered Cruller	270
Strawberry	210
Strawberry Frosted	210
Sugar Cruller	250
Sugar Raised	170
Sugar Cake	250
Toasted Coconut	300
Vanilla Frosted Coffee Roll	290
Vanilla Frosted	210
Vanilla Kreme Filled	270
Whole Wheat Glazed Cake	310

Munchkins

Cake, Butternut (3)	200
Cake, Chocolate Glazed (3)	200
Cake, Cinnamon (4)	250
Cake, Coconut (3)	200
Cake, Glazed (3)	200
Cake, Plain (4)	220
Cake, Powdered (4)	250
Cake, Sugared (4)	240
Cake, Toasted Coconut (3)	200
Yeast, Glazed (5)	200
Yeast, Jelly Filled (5)	210
Yeast, Lemon Filled (4)	170
Yeast, Sugar Raised (7)	220

Bagels, 1

Berry Berry	340
Blueberry	340
Cinnamon Raisin	340
Everything	360
Garlic	360
Onion	350
Plain	340
Poppyseed	360
Salsa Bagel	340
Salt	340
Sesame	380
Wheat	350

Muffins, Danish, Other

Danish, Apple	250
Danish, Cheese	270
Danish, Strawberry Cheese	250
Muffin, Banana Nut	530
Muffin, Blueberry	490
Muffin, Chocolate Chip	590
Muffin, Coffee Cake	710
Muffin, Corn	500
Muffin, Cranberry Orange	470
Muffin, Honey Bran Raisin	480
Muffin, Reduced Fat Blueberry	450

DUNKIN DONUTS – EINSTEIN BROTHERS BAGEL

Scone, Blueberry	410
Scone, Maple Walnut	470
Scone, Raspberry White Chocolate	450
Cookies (1 cookie)	
Chocolate Chunk	220
Chocolate Chunk w/nuts	230
Chocolate w/white Chocolate Chunks	230
Oatmeal Raisin Pecan	220
Spreads, 1 Pack	
Chive	190
Garden Vegetable	180
Lite	130
Plain	200
Salmon	180
Shedd's Buttermatch Blend	80
Strawberry	180
Breakfast	
Bagel, Egg, Bacon, Cheese	490
Bagel, Egg, Sausage, Cheese	650
Bagel, Egg, Steak, Cheese	640
Biscuit, Egg, Cheese	380
Biscuit, Egg, Sausage, Cheese	590
Croissant, Egg, Ham, Cheese	440
English Muffin, Ham, Egg, Cheese	320

Einstein Brothers Bagel

Bagels	**Calories**
Asiago Cheese Bagel	360
Bagel, Lucky Green	320
Bagel, Power	410
Chocolate Chip Bagel	370
Chopped Garlic Bagel	380
Chopped Onion Bagel	330
Cinnamon Raisin Swirl Bagel	350
Cinnamon Sugar Bagel	330
Cranberry Bagel	350
Dark Pumpernickel Bagel	320
Egg Bagel	340
Everything Bagel	340
Honey Whole Wheat Bagel	320
Jalapeno Bagel	330
Mango Bagel	360
Marble Rye Bagel	340
Nutty Banana Bagel	360
Plain Bagel	320
Poppy Dip'd Bagel	350
Potato Bagel	350
Power Bagel w/Peanut Butter	750
Pumpkin Bagel	330
Salt Bagel	330

EINSTEIN BROTHERS BAGEL

Sesame Dip'd Bagel	380
Sun-Dried Tomato Bagel	320
Wild Blueberry Bagel	350

Top Shelf Bagels

Roasted Red Pepper & Pesto	410
Six-Cheese Bagel	390
Spicy Nacho Bagel	450
Spinach Florentine	410

Bread Specialty

Bagel Mini Shtick Corn Meal	170
Bagel Mini Shtick Sesame	180
Bagel Shtick, Asiago	450
Bagel Shtick, Cinnamon Sugar	570
Bagel Shtick, Everything	380
Bagel Shtick, Potato	350
Bagel Shtick, Sesame	420
Bagel Twist	220
Challah Roll	300
Cheese Pizza Focaccia	500
Flat Bread, Peanut Sesame	650
Flat Bread, Rosemary & Asiago	520
Margarita Focaccia	400
Pepperoni Pizza Focaccia	590

Specialty Coffee

Americano, Regular	1
Americano, Large	1
Café Latte, Medium	200
Cafe Latte, Regular	140
Caffe Latte Non-fat Large	180
Caffe Latte Non-fat Medium	140
Caffe Latte Non-fat, Regular	100
Cage Latte, Large	250
Cappuccino Medium	190
Cappuccino Non-fat, Regular	60
Cappuccino, Large	230
Cappuccino, Large (low-fat Milk)	150
Cappuccino, Medium (low-fat Milk)	130
Cappuccino, Regular	90
Chai 2% Milk, Large	340
Chai 2% Milk, Medium	270
Chai 2% Milk, Regular	210
Chai Skim Milk, Large	310
Chai Skim Milk, Medium	250
Chai Skim Milk, Regular	190
Espresso, Regular	1
Low Fat Mocha Large	420
Low Fat Mocha Medium	350
Low Fat Mocha, Regular	190
Mocha, Large	470
Mocha, Medium	390

Mocha, Regular	230
Iced Specialty Coffee	
Iced Americano, 8 oz	0
Iced Coffee, Regular	0
Iced Latte, Medium	120
Iced Mocha, Medium	210
Iced Non Fat Latte, Medium	90
Low Fat Iced Mocha, Medium	180
Low Fat Mocha, Regular	190
Coffee Extras (2 Tblsp)	
Light Whipped Cream	30
On Top Reduced Fat Topping	20
Syrups	
Syrup, Almond	90
Syrup, Hazelnut	80
Syrup, Premium, Sugar Free Caramel	0
Syrup, Premium, Sugar Free Vanilla	0
Syrup, Raspberry	80
Syrup, Vanilla	80
Cold Beverages	
Apple Juice Box	120
Fruit Punch Juice Box	90
Half & Half	40
Iced Tea, Unsweetened	0
Low Fat 2% Milk	120
Minute Maid Country Style OJ	100
Minute Maid Orange	106
Minute Maid Orig. Style Lemonade	96
Minute Maid Premium Orange Juice	110
Nestea Peach Iced Tea	78
Nestea Raspberry Iced Tea	78
Nestea Southern Style Iced Tea	123
Nestea Unsweetened Iced Tea	0
Odwalla Fresh Squeezed Orange Juice	143
Smoothie, Mocha	470
Condiments	
Ancho Lime Mayo (1 Tblsp)	50
Ancho Lime Salsa (1/4 Cup)	20
Deli Mustard (1 tsp)	4
French Dijon Mustard (1 tsp)	10
Grained Dijon Mustard (1 tsp)	5
Honey Mustard (1 tsp)	15
Marinated Red Onions (4 oz)	150
Raspberry Mustard (2 Tblsp)	50
Whole Kosher Pickle (1)	5
Yellow Mustard (1 Tblsp)	0
Cream Cheese (2 Tblsp)	
Whipped Blueberry	70
Whipped Cappuccino	70
Whipped Garden Vegetable	60

EINSTEIN BROTHERS BAGEL

Whipped Honey Almond Red. Fat	70
Whipped Jalapeno Salsa	60
Whipped Maple Raisin Walnut	60
Whipped Onion And Chive	70
Whipped Plain	70
Whipped Plain Reduced Fat	60
Whipped Pumpkin	100
Whipped Smoked Salmon	60
Whipped Strawberry	70
Whipped Sun Dried Tomato & Basil	60

Hot Tea

Cinnamon Apple Spice	0
Earl Grey	0
English Breakfast	0
Lemon Zinger	0
Mandarin Orange Spice	0
Peppermint	0

Other Hot Beverages

Hot Chocolate, Regular	290
Lower Fat Hot Chocolate, Regular	260

Retail, Food

Fruit and Yogurt Parfait	190
Kettle Classic Natural Potato Chips	100
Tortilla Strips	140

Roll-Ups

Albuquerque Turkey	790
Thai Vegetable	630
Thai Vegetable w/Chicken	670

Salad Dressings

Asian Sesame Dressing	80
Caesar Dressing	150
Chipotle BBQ Dressing	110
Honey Chipotle Dressing	140
Horseradish Sauce Dressing	170
Raspberry Vinaigrette Dressing	160
Thousand Island	110
Wasabi Oriental Dressing	80

Salad Extras

Bagel Croutons	25
Sweet Roasted Walnuts	180

Salads

Asian Chicken Salad	550
Bros Bistro	520
Caesar Salad	650
Chicken Caesar Salad	750
Chicken Chipotle Salad	710
Chicken Salad On Greens	210
Egg Salad	200
Fresh Fruit Cup	110
Mixed Greens	220

EINSTEIN BROTHERS BAGEL

Roasted Corn Salad	90
Traditional Potato Salad	290
Tuna Salad	150
Tuna Salad On Greens	170
Sandwich Fillings	
American Cheese (1 slice)	70
Bacon, Peppered (3 slices)	90
Cheddar Cheese (1 slice)	80
Cheese, Pepper Jack (1 slice)	100
Provolone Cheese (1 slice)	70
Smoked Salmon, Port Chatham (2 oz)	110
Smoked Salmon, Sea Specialties (2 oz)	92
Swiss Cheese (1 Slice)	80
Sandwich, Assembled	
Chicago Bagel Dog (onion, no cheese)	680
Chicago Bagel Dog, Asiago	740
Chicago Bagel Dog, Everything	730
Chicago Chili Cheese Bagel Dog	810
Chicken Salad	500
Egg Salad	560
Egg, Homeststyle Bacon	580
Egg, Homestyle Ham	530
Egg, Homestyle Sausage	550
Egg, Original	480
Egg, Salmon and Shmear	650
Egg, Santa Fe	650
Ham	450
Holey Cow	900
Hummus & Feta	540
New York Lox & Bagels	660
Roast Beef	460
Rueben Deli	660
Smoked Turkey	420
Tasty Turkey	570
The Veg Out	490
Tuna Salad	470
Turkey Pastrami Deli	440
Bread Sandwiches On 12 Grain	
Deli Chicken Salad	440
Deli Egg Salad	490
Deli Ham	560
Deli Roast Beef	560
Deli Smoked Turkey	530
Deli Tuna Salad	440
Deli Turkey Pastrami	540
Ultimate Toasted Cheese w/ Tomato	870
Bread Sandwiches On Country White	
Deli Chicken Salad	540
Deli Egg Salad	590
Deli Ham	660

EINSTEIN BROTHERS BAGEL

Deli Roast Beef	660
Deli Smoked Turkey	630
Deli Tuna Salad	510
Deli Turkey Pastrami	640
Ultimate Toasted Cheese w/ Tomato	870

Challah Deli Sandwiches

Club Mex	750
Cobbie	630
Deli Chicken Salad	480
Deli Egg Salad	430
Deli Pastrami	480
Deli Roast Beef	500
Deli Smoked Turkey	470
Deli Tuna Salad	370
Deli Turkey Ham	500
EBBQ Chicken Sandwich	380
Roasted Chicken & Smoked Gouda	440

Panini's

Cali Club Panini	730
Cuban Ham Panini	700
Italian Chicken Panini	770
Taos Turkey Panini	740
Ultimate Toasted Cheese Panini	900

Soups

Broccoli, Sharp Cheddar (Bowl)	540
Broccoli, Sharp Cheddar (Cup)	230
Chicken & Wild Rice (Bowl)	440
Chicken & Wild Rice (Cup)	190
Chicken Noodle (Bowl)	510
Chicken Noodle (Cup)	220
Clam Chowder (Bowl)	370
Clam Chowder (Cup)	160
Low Fat Minestrone (Bowl)	430
Low Fat Minestrone (Cup)	180
Tomato Bisque (Bowl)	440
Tomato Bisque (Cup)	190
Tortilla Soup (Bowl)	200
Tortilla Soup (Cup)	90
Turkey Chili (Cup)	140
Turkey Chili Bowl	330

Spreads

Butter (1 Tblsp)	100
Butter and Margarine Blend Spread (1 Tblsp)	60
Fruit Spread, Apricot (1 oz)	75
Fruit Spread, Grape (1 oz)	75
Fruit Spread, Strawberry (1 oz)	75
Honey Butter (1 Tblsp)	90
Hummus, Retail (12oz)	110
Peanut Butter, Creamy (2 Tblsp)	190

EINSTEIN BROTHERS BAGEL

Choose Two

Half Salads

Asian Chicken	234
Bros. Bistro	272
Caesar Side	220
Roasted Chicken Caesar	267

Half Sandwiches On Bagel

Half Ham	227
Half Harvest Chicken Salad	274
Half Holy Cow	453
Half Hummus And Feta	279
Half N.Y. Lox And Bagel	338
Half Roast Beef	234
Half Smoked Turkey	213
Half Tasty Turkey	304
Half Tuna Salad	256
Half Turkey Pastrami	225
Half Turkey Pastrami Rueben	338
Half Veg Out	255

Half Sandwiches On 12 Grain

Half Chicken Salad	244
Half Egg Salad	251
Half Ham	364
Half Roast Beef	288
Half Smoked Turkey	275
Half Tuan Salad	213
Half Turkey Pastrami	279
Half Ultimate Toasted Cheese	453

Half Sandwiches On Country White

Half Chicken Salad	338
Half Egg Salad	308
Half Ham	346
Half Roast Beef	345
Half Smoked Turkey	316
Half Tuna Salad	270
Half Turkey Pastrami	336
Half Ultimate Toasted Cheese	454

Half Challah Sandwiches

Half Chicken Salad	211
Half Club Mex	383
Half Cobbie	321
Half EBBQ Chicken Sandwich	196
Half Egg Salad	218
Half Ham	265
Half Pastrami	255
Half Roast Beef	264
Half Roasted Chicken & Smoked Gouda	231
Half Smoked Turkey	251
Half Tuna Salad	189

EINSTEIN BROTHERS BAGEL – FAZOLI'S

Sweets

Banana Nut Muffin	580
Blueberry Figure 8	390
Blueberry Muffin	480
Blueberry Scone w/icing	450
Cherry Figure 8	400
Chocolate Chip Muffin	590
Chocolate Chunk Cookie	640
Cinnamon Roll	810
Cinnamon Walnut Strudel	550
Ginger White Chocolate Cookie	510
Iced Brownie	550
Iced Brownie w/walnuts	600
Lemon Currant Scone	430
Oatmeal Raisin Cookie	600
Peanut Butter Cookie	640
Pound Cake, Lemon Iced (1 slice)	540
Pound Cake, Marble (1 slice)	460
Pumpkin Pecan Muffin	480
Rice Krispy Bars (1 Bar)	420
Sweetie Pie	620

LTO Seasonal Products

Black Forrest Muffin	510
Caramel Apple Latte Large Low-Fat	270
Caramel Apple Latte Large Skim	220
Caramel Apple Latte Med Low Fat	230
Caramel Apple Latte Med Skim	190
Caramel Apple Latte Reg Low-Fat	170
Caramel Apple Latte Reg Skim	140
Chocolate Truffle Cookie	510
Eggnog Latte Large	530
Eggnog Latte Med	400
Eggnog Latte Reg	320
Hashbrowns Stack	150
Orange Mango Bagel	360
Peach Mango Muffin	450
Pumpkin Bagel	330
Pumpkin Cream Cheese	100
Pumpkin Pecan Muffin	480
Pumpkin White Chocolate Spice Cookie	389
Seasonal Sugar Cookie	450
White Chocolate Lemon Iced Cookie	510
White Chocolate Macaroon	170

Fazoli's

Italian Specialties	Calories
Baked Chicken Alfredo	790
Baked Chicken Parmesan	740
Baked Spaghetti Parmesan	700
Baked Ziti	490

FAZOLI'S

Baked Ziti - Regular	750
Broccoli Fettuccine Alfredo - Regular	830
Broccoli Lasagna	750
Cheese Ravioli w/Marinara	480
Cheese Ravioli w/Meat Sauce	510
Classic Sampler	830
Homestyle Lasagna w/Meat Sauce	680
Pizza Baked Spaghetti	750
Shrimp & Scallop Fettuccine	610

Pastas

Broccoli Fettuccine Alfredo	560
Fettuccine Alfredo	530
Fettuccine Alfredo-Regular	800
Peppery Chicken Alfredo	610
Spaghetti w/Marinara	420
Spaghetti w/Marinara-Regular	620
Spaghetti w/Meat Sauce	450
Spaghetti w/Meat Sauce-Regular	670
Spaghetti w/Meatballs	720
Spaghetti w/Meatballs-Regular	1020

Pizza

Cheese Pizza - Double Slice	460
Combination Pizza - Double Slice	570
Pepperoni Pizza - Double Slice	530

Breadsticks

1 Breadstick	140
1 Breadstick - Dry	90

Submarinos & Paninis

Chicken Caesar Club Panini	660
Chicken Pesto Panini	510
Four Cheese & Tomato Panini	720
Ham & Swiss Panini	600
Italian Club Panini	670
Italian Deli Panini	660
Smoked Turkey Panini	710
Submarino Club - Half	1100
Submarino Ham & Swiss - Half	1000
Submarino Meatball - Half	1260
Submarino Original - Half	1160
Submarino Pepperoni Pizza - Half	1060
Submarino Turkey - Half	990

Soups and Salads

Chicken & Pasta Caesar Salad	370
Chicken Caesar Salad	420
Chicken Finger Salad	190
Chicken Finger Salad w/Bacon Honey Mustard Dressing	400
Garden Salad	30
Italian Chef Salad	260
Minestrone Soup	120
Pasta Salad	590

FAZOLI'S – GODFATHER'S PIZZA

Side Pasta Salad	240
Dressings	
Honey French Dressing	150
House Italian Dressing	110
Ranch Dressing	150
Reduced Calorie Italian Dressing	50
Thousand Island Dressing	130
Desserts	
Cheesecake - Chocolate Chip	300
Cheesecake - Plain	290
Cheesecake - Turtle	420
Lemon Ice	190
Milk Chocolate Chunk Cookie	360
Strawberry Topping	35

Freshen's

Smoothies	Calories
Aruba Orange	420
Blueberry Sunset	385
Blueberry Wave	330
Caribbean Craze	330
Coffee, Caramel	430
Coffee, Mocha	375
Coffee, Original	340
Fudge Supreme	645
Jamaican Jammer	475
Orange Shooter	375
Orange Surprise	415
Orange Wave	420
Peach Sunset	365
Peachy Pineapple	405
Peanut Butter Cup	935
Pina Collider	560
Pineapple Passion	420
Raspberry Rapture	515
Raspberry Rhapsody	345
Raspberry Rocker	490
Raspberry Rumba	375
Strawberry Shooter	245
Strawberry Squeeze	390

Godfather's Pizza

Mini-Original Crust (4 slices)	Calories
All Meat Combo	880
Bacon Cheeseburger	860
Cheese	600
Combo	830
Hawaiian	650
Pepperoni	650

Taco	830
Veggie	640
Medium-Original (1 slice)	
All Meat Combo	370
Bacon Cheeseburger	330
Cheese	260
Combo	350
Hawaiian	280
Pepperoni	290
Taco	350
Veggie	280
Large-Original (1 slice)	
All Meat Combo	410
Bacon Cheeseburger	400
Cheese	290
Combo	390
Hawaiian	320
Pepperoni	330
Taco	410
Veggie	310
Jumbo-Original (1 slice)	
All Meat Combo	610
Bacon Cheeseburger	590
Cheese	430
Combo	580
Hawaiian	460
Pepperoni	490
Taco	580
Veggie	460
Medium-Golden Crust (1 slice)	
All Meat Combo	300
Bacon Cheeseburger	240
Cheese	220
Combo	290
Hawaiian	240
Pepperoni	260
Taco	290
Veggie	230
Large-Golden Crust (1 slice)	
All Meat Combo	350
Bacon Cheeseburger	330
Cheese	250
Combo	330
Hawaiian	270
Pepperoni	290
Taco	340
Veggie	260
Medium-Thin Crust (1 slice)	
All Meat Combo	280

GODFATHER'S PIZZA – HAAGEN-DAZS

Bacon Cheeseburger	250
Cheese	200
Combo	270
Hawaiian	220
Pepperoni	230
Taco	270
Veggie	210

Large-Thin Crust (1 slice)

All Meat Combo	310
Bacon Cheeseburger	290
Cheese	220
Combo	290
Hawaiian	230
Pepperoni	250
Taco	300
Veggie	230

Haagen-Dazs

Ice Cream (1/2 Cup)	Calories
Baileys Irish Cream	270
Bananas Foster	260
Belgian Chocolate	330
Blueberry Cheesecake	310
Butter Pecan	310
Café Mocha Frappe	310
Cherry Vanilla	240
Chocolate	270
Chocolate Brownie & Walnuts	290
Chocolate Caramel	320
Chocolate Cheesecake	300
Chocolate Chocolate Chip	300
Chocolate Cookies & Cream	270
Chocolate Mousse	310
Chocolate Peanut Butter	360
Chocolate Raspberry Torte	270
Coffee	270
Coffee Almond Swirl	320
Cookie Dough Chip	310
Cookies & Cream	270
Crème Brulee	280
Crème Caramel Pecan	320
Dulche De Leche	290
French Vanilla Mousse	310
German Chocolate Cake	290
Macadamia Brittle	300
Mango	250
Mint Chip	300
Mocha Almond Fudge	340
Peanut Butter Fudge Chunk	340

Pecan Pie	330
Pineapple Coconut	230
Pistachio	290
Pralines & Cream	290
Rocky Road	300
Rum Raisin	270
Strawberry	240
Strawberry Cheesecake	270
Tres Leches	290
Vanilla	270
Vanilla Caramel Brownie	300
Vanilla Cherry Fudge Chunk	310
Vanilla Chocolate Chip	310
Vanilla Fudge	290
Vanilla Fudge Brownie	300
Vanilla Swiss Almond	300
Sorbet (1/2 Cup)	
All Other Flavors	120
Orchard Peach	130
Gelato (1/2 Cup)	
Cappuccino	240
Chocolate	240
Hazelnut	260
Raspberry	240
Frozen Yogurt (1/2 Cup)	
Apple Pie	230
Banana Cream Pie	220
Chocolate Fudge Brownie	190
Coffee	200
Dulche De Leche	190
Lemon Pie	260
Peach Melba	210
Pumpkin Cheesecake	240
Strawberry	140
Strawberry Cheesecake	230
Vanilla	200
Vanilla Raspberry Swirl	170
Bars (1 Bar)	
Caramel & Almond Crunch	310
Caramel & Pecan Nut Cluster	420
Chocolate & Dark Chocolate	350
Chocolate Fudge & Almonds	330
Chocolate Sorbet	80
Coffee & Almond Crunch	370
Cookies & Cream Crunch	370
Dulche De Leche	300
Raspberry Cheesecake	310
Raspberry Sorbet & Vanilla Yogurt	90
Tres Leches	290

HAAGEN-DAZS – HARDEE'S

Vanilla & Almonds	380
Vanilla & Dark Chocolate	280
Vanilla & Milk Chocolate	340
Vanilla Caramel & Pecans	350

Hardee's

Chicken	Calories
Chicken Strips (3)	120
Chicken Strips (5)	200
Fried Chicken Breast	370
Fried Chicken Leg	170
Fried Chicken Thigh	330
Fried Chicken Wing	200

Sides

Cole Slaw (Small)	240
Crispy Curls™ Potatoes (Large)	590
Crispy Curls™ Potatoes (Medium)	520
Crispy Curls™ Potatoes (Small)	340
French Fries (Large)	510
French Fries (Medium)	440
French Fries (Small)	340
Gravy	20
Mashed Potatoes (Small)	70

Burgers & Sandwiches

1/2 lb Grilled Sourdough	1010
1/2 lb Six Dollar	900
1/3 lb Bacon Cheese	800
1/3 lb Cheeseburger	615
1/3 lb Chili Cheese	855
1/3 lb Thickburger	740
2/3 lb Double Bacon Cheese	1150
2/3 lb Double Thickburger	1090
BBQ Grilled Chicken Sandwich	270
Big Hot Ham 'N' Cheese	445
Big Roast Beef™ Sandwich	395
Cheeseburger	315
Chicken Filet Sandwich	435
Famous Star™	550
Fisherman's Filet™ Sandwich	520
Frisco® Burger	725
Hamburger	265
Hot Dog	450
Hot Ham 'N' Cheese™ Sandwich	305
Monster Burger®	950
Regular Roast Beef Sandwich	310
Slammer	270
Slammer w/Cheese	320
Super Star®	640
The Six Dollar Burger™	910

Breakfast

Apple Cinnamon 'N' Raisin™ Biscuit	250
Bacon, Egg & Cheese Biscuit	521
Biscuit 'N' Gravy™	530
Chicken Biscuit	540
Cinnamon 'N' Raisin™ Biscuit	250
Cinnamon Roll	535
Country Ham Biscuit	434
Frisco® Breakfast Sandwich	456
Ham Biscuit	410
Jelly Biscuit	440
Made from Scratch® Biscuit (No Margarine)	360
Made from Scratch® Biscuit (w/Margarine)	390
Omelette™ Biscuit	550
Regular Hash Rounds™ Potatoes (16)	230
Sausage & Egg Biscuit	621
Sausage & Egg Biscuit	621
Sausage Biscuit	553
Steak Biscuit	576

Dessert

Apple Turnover	270
Chocolate Chip Cookie	370
Peach Cobbler (Small)	310
Twist Cone	180

Drinks

Chocolate Shake	370
Hot Chocolate	120
Iced Tea	5
Orange Juice, 10 oz.	140
Raspberry Nestea® (Small)	160
Vanilla Shake	350

In-N-Out Burger

Burgers	Calories
Hamburger	390
w/Mustard & Ketchup, No Spread	310
Protein Style, No Buns, Lettuce	240
Cheeseburger	480
w/Mustard & Ketchup, No Spread	400
Protein Style, No Buns, Lettuce	330
Double-Double®	670
w/Mustard & Ketchup, No Spread	590
Protein Style, No Buns, Lettuce	520

Sides

French Fries	400
Chocolate Shake	690
Strawberry Shake	690
Vanilla Shake	680

Drinks

Coffee	5

IN-N-OUT BURGER – KFC

Iced Tea	0
Lemonade	180
Milk	180
Root Beer	222

Jamba Juice

Smoothies (24 oz.)	Calories
Aloha Pineapple	470
Banana Berry	470
Berry Lime Sublime	590
Bounce Back Blast	480
Caribbean Passion	440
Chocolate Moo'd	690
Citrus Squeeze	450
Coldbuster	430
Cranberry Craze	420
Jamba Powerboost	440
Kiwi Berry Burner	470
Mango-A-Go-Go	500
Orange Dream Machine	540
Orange-A-Peel	440
Orange Berry Blitz	410
Peach Pleasure	460
Peanut Butter Moo'd	860
Peenya Kowlada	650
Protein Berry Pizzazz	440
Razzmatazz	480
Strawberries Wild	450
Strawberry Dream'n	470
Juices (16 oz.)	
Carrot	100
Lemonade	300
Orange	220
Orange/Banana	220
Orange/Carrot	160
Vibrant-C	210
Wheatgrass (1 oz)	5
Baked Goods	
Apple Cinnamon Pretzel	420
Grin'n'Carrot	250
Honey Berry Bran	320
Lemon Poppyseed Bundt	300
Pizza Protein Stick	230
Sourdough Parmesan Pretzel	460

KFC

Chicken	Calories
Chicken Pot Pie	770
Extra Crispy - Breast	470

KFC

Extra Crispy - Drumstick	160
Extra Crispy - Thigh	370
Extra Crispy Whole Wing	190
Hot & Spicy - Breast	450
Hot & Spicy - Drumstick	140
Hot & Spicy - Thigh	390
Hot & Spicy - Whole Wing	180
Original - Breast	370
Original - Drumstick	140
Original - Thigh	360
Original - Whole Wing	145
Popcorn Chicken, Large	620
Popcorn Chicken, Small	360
Strips, Blazin' (3)	315
Strips, Colonels (3)	340
Strips, Honey BBQ (3)	375
Strips, Spicy Crispy (3)	335
Wings, Honey BBQ (6)	605
Wings, Hot Wings (6)	470

Sandwiches

Honey BBQ Crunch Melt	550
Honey BBQ Flavor	310
Original Recipe no sauce	360
Original Recipe w/sauce	450
Tender Roast no sauce	270
Tender Roast w/sauce	350
Triple Crunch no sauce	390
Triple Crunch w/Sauce	490
Triple Crunch Zinger no sauce	390
Triple Crunch Zinger w/sauce	550
Twister	600
Twister, Blazin'	720
Twister, Crispy Caesar	745

Sides

BBQ Baked Beans	190
Biscuit (1)	180
Cole Slaw	235
Corn On The Cob	150
Green Beans	45
Macaroni & Cheese	180
Mashed Potatoes w/gravy	120
Mean Greens	70
Potato Salad	230
Potato Wedges	375

Desserts

Double Chocolate Chip Cake	320
Parfait, Chocolate Crème	290
Parfait, Fudge Brownie	280
Parfait, Lemon Crème	410
Parfait, Strawberry Shortcake	200

KFC – KRISPY KREME

Pie, Apple (1 slice)	310
Pie, Pecan (1 slice)	490
Pie, Strawberry Creme (1 slice)	280

Krispy Kreme

Yeast DoughNuts	**Calories**
Chocolate Iced Glazed	250
Chocolate Iced Glazed w/Sprinkles	260
Cinnamon Bun	260
Cinnamon Twist	230
Cranapple Crunch Filled	330
Dulche De Leche (Filled)	290
Glazed	200
Glazed Cinnamon	210
Glazed Pumpkin Spice	340
Glazed Twist	210
Maple Iced Glazed	250
Sugar	200
Cake DoughNuts	
Chocolate Iced Glazed Cruller	280
Chocolate Mini-cake	270
Glazed Cruller	240
Glazed, Blueberry	300
Glazed, Devil's Food	340
Honey & Oat	270
Plain Mini-cake	250
Powdered Sugar	260
Powdered Sugar Mini-cake	210
Sour Cream	280
Traditional	220
Traditional, Chocolate Iced	270
Vanilla Iced w/Sprinkles	280
Filled DoughNuts	
Apple Filled, Cinnamon Sugar Coated	280
Blueberry Filled, Powdered Sugar Coated	270
Chocolate Iced Crème Filled	340
Chocolate Iced Custard Filled	310
Glazed Cherry Filled	290
Glazed Crème Filled	350
Glazed Raspberry Filled	350
Yeast - Glazed Custard Filled	290
Yeast - Glazed Lemon Filled	290
Yeast - Powdered Raspberry Filled	300
Yeast - Powdered Strawberry Filled	260
Yeast - Vanilla Iced Crème Filled	360
Yeast - Vanilla Iced Custard Filled	290
Other Items	
Apple Pie	400
Cherry Pie	410
Chocolate Enrobed Doughnut Holes	270

KRISPY KREME – LITTLE CEASAR'S

Coconut Crème Pie	450
Glazed Doughnut Holes	220
Glazed Mini-Cruller	230
Honey Bun	410
Peach Pie	370
Powdered Sugar Doughnut Holes	220
Original Kreme	270
Original Kreme w/Coffee	245
Raspberry	350
Frozen Beverages	
Double Fudge	320
Double Fudge w/Coffee	320
Latte	250

Krystal

Item	Calories
Apple Turnover	220
Biscuit, Bacon, Egg, & Cheese	390
Biscuit, Chik	340
Biscuit, Plain	260
Biscuit, Sausage	440
Chili	200
Corn Pup	260
Country Breakfast	660
Fries, Chili Cheese	540
Fries, Reg	370
Hash Browns	190
Krystal	160
Krystal Chik	240
Krystal, Bacon Cheese	190
Krystal, Cheese	180
Krystal, Double	260
Krystal, Double Cheese	310
Lemon Meringue Pie	360
Pup, Chili Cheese	210
Pup, Plain	170
Sunriser	240

Little Ceasar's

Pizza By The Slice	Calories
12″ Round Pizza (1 slice)	
Cheese Only	167
Pepperoni	190
14″ Round Pizza (1 slice)	
Cheese Only	180
Pepperoni	204
Supreme	257
Meat	285
Veggie	199

LITTLE CEASAR'S – LONG JOHN SILVERS

12" Thin Crust (1 slice)

Cheese Only	141
Pepperoni	150

14" Thin Crust (1 slice)

Cheese Only	140
Pepperoni	164

16" Round Pizza (1 slice)

Cheese Only	193
Pepperoni	220

18" Round Pizza (1 slice)

Cheese Only	213
Pepperoni	268

12" DeepDish (Square) 1 slice

Cheese Only	206
Pepperoni	233

14" DeepDish (Square) 1 Slice

Cheese Only	280
Pepperoni	312

Pizza By The Slice (1/6 of a 14")

Cheese Only	301
Pepperoni	348

Sides

Baby Pan! Pan!	363
Chicken Wings (1 wing)	53
Cinnamon Crazy Sticks	63
Crazy Bread (1 stick)	98
Crazy Sauce	45
Italian Cheese Bread (1 piece)	124

Cold Sandwiches

Deli Italian	690
Deli Veggie	720
Deli Ham and Cheese	600

Salads

Tossed Side	50
Antipasto	175

Dressings

Italian	200
Ranch	221
Fat-free Italian	15

Long John Silvers

Item (1 Piece/Sandwich)	Calories
Battered Chicken	130
Battered Clams	240
Battered Fish	230
Battered Shrimp	45
Chicken Sandwich	340
Fish Sandwich	440
Ultimate Fish Sandwich	480

Sides & Starters

Cheese sticks (3)	140
Clam Chowder (1 bowl)	220
Cole Slaw	200
Corn Cobbette (1)	90
Crumblies	170
Fries, Large	390
Fries, Reg	230
Hushpuppies (1)	60
Rice	180

Desserts

Chocolate Cream Pie	310
Pecan Pie	370
Pineapple Cream Pie	290

McDonald's

Sandwiches	Calories
Big Mac®	590
Big N' Tasty®	530
Big N' Tasty® w/Cheese	580
Cheeseburger	330
Chicken McGrill®	400
Crispy Chicken	500
Double Cheeseburger	480
Double Quarter Pounder® w/Cheese	760
Filet-O-Fish®	470
Grilled Chicken FlatBread	520
Hamburger	280
Hot 'n Spicy McChicken®	450
McChicken®	430
Quarter Pounder® w/Cheese	530
Quarter Pounder®	420

French Fries

Small French Fries	210
McValue® French Fries	320
Medium French Fries	450
Large French Fries	540
Super Size® French Fries	610

Chicken McNuggets/Sauces

Chicken McNuggets® (4 Piece)	210
Chicken McNuggets® (6 Piece)	310
Chicken McNuggets® (10 Piece)	510
Chicken McNuggets® (20 Piece)	1030
Barbeque Sauce	45
Honey	45
Honey Mustard Sauce	50
Hot Mustard Sauce	60
Light Mayonnaise	45
Sweet 'N Sour Sauce	50

MCDONALD'S

Salads

Bacon Ranch (without chicken)	140
Butter Garlic Croutons	50
Caesar (without chicken)	90
California Cobb (without chicken)	160
Crispy Chicken Bacon Ranch	370
Crispy Chicken Caesar Salad	310
Crispy Chicken California Cobb	380
Grilled Chicken Bacon Ranch	270
Grilled Chicken Caesar	210
Grilled Chicken California Cobb	280
Side	15

Salad Dressings

Newman's Own® Cobb	120
Newman's Own® Creamy Caesar	190
Newman's Own® Light Balsamic Vinaigrette	90
Newman's Own® Ranch	290

Breakfast

Bacon, Egg & Cheese Biscuit	480
Bacon, Egg & Cheese McGriddles™	450
Bagel (Plain)	260
Big Breakfast	710
Biscuit	240
Cinnamon Roll	340
Egg McMuffin®	300
English Muffin	150
Ham, Egg & Cheese Bagel	550
Hash Browns	130
Hotcakes (margarine 2 pats & syrup)	600
Sausage	170
Sausage Biscuit	410
Sausage Biscuit w/egg	490
Sausage Breakfast Burrito	290
Sausage McGriddles™	420
Sausage McMuffin®	370
Sausage McMuffin® w/Egg	450
Sausage, Egg & Cheese McGriddles™	550
Scrambled Eggs (2)	160
Spanish Omelette Bagel	710
Steak, Egg & Cheese Bagel	640

Desserts/Shakes

Baked Apple Pie	260
Butterfinger® McFlurry™ (12 oz)	620
Butterfinger® McFlurry™ (16 oz)	900
Chocolate Chip Cookie	170
Chocolate Shake (12 fl oz Cup)	430
Chocolate Shake (16 fl oz Cup)	580
Chocolate Shake (21 fl oz Cup)	750
Chocolate Shake (32 fl oz Cup)	1150
Fruit 'n Yogurt Parfait	380

MCDONALD'S – MIAMI SUBS

Fruit 'n Yogurt Parfait (w/o Granola)	280
Hot Caramel Sundae	360
Hot Fudge Sundae	340
Kiddie Cone	45
M&M® McFlurry™ (12 fl oz Cup)	630
M&M® McFlurry™ (16 fl oz Cup)	910
McDonaldland® Chocolate Chip Cookies	280
McDonaldland® Cookies	230
Nestle Crunch® McFlurry® (12 fl oz Cup)	630
Nestle Crunch® McFlurry® (16 fl oz Cup)	920
Nuts (for Sundaes)	40
Oreo® McFlurry™ (12 fl oz Cup)	570
Oreo® McFlurry™ (16 fl oz Cup)	820
Snack Size Fruit 'n Yogurt Parfait	160
Snack Size Fruit 'n Yogurt Parfait (w/o granola)	130
Strawberry Shake (12 fl oz Cup)	420
Strawberry Shake (16 fl oz Cup)	560
Strawberry Shake (21 fl oz Cup)	730
Strawberry Shake (32 fl oz Cup)	1120
Strawberry Sundae	290
Vanilla Reduced Fat Ice Cream Cone	150
Vanilla Shake (12 fl oz Cup)	430
Vanilla Shake (16 fl oz Cup)	570
Vanilla Shake (21 fl oz Cup)	750
Vanilla Shake (32 fl oz Cup)	1140

Beverages

1% low-fat Milk	100
Coffee (Large)	0
Coffee (Medium)	0
Coffee (Small)	0
Half & Half® Creamer	15
Iced Tea	0
Orange Juice (12 fl oz Cup)	140
Orange Juice (16 fl oz Cup)	180
Orange Juice (21 fl oz Cup)	250

Miami Subs

Cheesesteak 6"	Calories
Chicken Philly Classic	550
Classic	420
Original	410
Works	530
Subs 6"	
Ham & Cheese	450
Italian Deli	515
Meatball	490
Tuna	470
Turkey	485
Burgers	
Deluxe	785

MIAMI SUBS – MRS. FIELDS

Deluxe Bacon Cheeseburger	920
Deluxe Cheeseburger	860
Pitas	
Chicken Pita	390
Gyros Pita	660
Platters	
Chicken Breast Platter	740
Gyros Platter	1420
10 Wings, Fries, Celery, Blue Cheese	1020
Salads	
Caesar w/dressing	460
Chicken Caesar w/dressing	610
Chicken Club	490
Garden	310
Greek	285
Greek Side w/dressing	79
Sides	
Fries, Large	1040
Fries, Regular	530
Mozzarella Sticks	755
Onion Rings	870

Mrs. Fields

Cookies	Calories
Butter Toffee	290
Cinnamon Sugar	300
Coconut & Macadamias	280
Debra's Special	280
Milk Chocolate & Walnuts	320
Milk Chocolate without nuts	280
Oatmeal Chocolate Chip	280
Oatmeal, Raisins and Walnuts	180
Peanut Butter	310
Peanut Butter Milk Chocolate	300
Semi-Sweet Chocolate	280
Semi-Sweet Chocolate w/Walnuts	310
Snickerdoodle Jumbo Cookie	640
White Chunk Macadamia	310
Bundt Cakes	
Banana Walnut	350
Banana Walnut w/Chocolate Chips	370
Blueberry	270
Raspberry	270
White Cake w/Chocolate Chips	350
Brownies	
Double Fudge	360
Frosted Fudge	440
Pecan Fudge	340
Pecan Pie Brownie	340
Walnut Fudge	380

MRS. FIELDS – OLD SPAGHETTI FACTORY

Bite-Size Nibbler® Cookies

Butter	110
Chewy Chocolate Fudge	110
Cinnamon Sugar	120
Milk Chocolate	110
Milk Chocolate w/Walnuts	120
Peanut Butter	110
Semi-Sweet Chocolate	110
Triple Chocolate	110
White Chunk Macadamia	120

Nathan's Famous

Item	Calories
1/4 lb Burger	535
1/4 lb Burger w/Cheese	850
Bacon Cheeseburger	705
Cheesesteak, Chicken	565
Cheesesteak, Original	740
Cheesesteak, Supreme	785
Fish Sandwich	470
Fries, Large	760
Fries, Regular	545
Fries, Super	1190
Hot Dog	310
Hot Dog Nuggets (6)	350
Onion Rings, Large	745
Onion Rings, Small	560
Super Burger	865

Old Spaghetti Factory

Item	Calories
Baked Lasagna	590
Chicken Marsala	1110
Chicken Parmigiana	630
Fettuccine Alfredo	1140
Spaghetti Pot Pourri	990
Spaghetti w/Clam Sauce	720
Spaghetti w/Clam/Meat Sauce	620
Spaghetti w/Clam/Mushroom Sauce	580
Spaghetti w/Meat Sauce	520
Spaghetti w/Meatballs/Tomato Sauce	720
Spaghetti w/Mizithra Cheese	910
Spaghetti w/Mizithra/Clam Sauce	810
Spaghetti w/Mizithra/Meat Sauce	720
Spaghetti w/Mizithra/Mushroom Sauce	680
Spaghetti w/Mizithra/Tomato Sauce	670
Spaghetti w/Mushroom Sauce	450
Spaghetti w/Mushroom/Meat Sauce	490
Spaghetti w/Mushroom/Tomato Sauce	450

OLD SPAGHETTI FACTORY - PANERA BREAD

Spaghetti w/Sausage/Meat Sauce	730
Spaghetti w/Tomato Sauce	440
Spaghetti w/Tomato/Clam Sauce	570
Spaghetti w/Tomato/Meat Sauce	480
Spinach & Cheese Ravioli	650
Spinach Tortellini w/Alfredo Sauce	1180
Salad Dressing	
Thousand Island, 1.5 oz	180
Balsamic Vinaigrette, 1 oz	160
Blue Cheese, 1.5 oz	200
Caesar, 1.5 oz	270
Creamy Pesto, 1.5 oz	210
Honey Mustard, 2 Tblsp	40

Olive Garden

Garden Fare Menu	**Calories**
Dinner Selection	< 600
Lunch Selection	< 400

Panera Bread

Bagels	**Calories**
Asiago Cheese	330
Blueberry	330
Cinnamon Crunch	510
Dutch Apple & Raisin	350
Everything	300
French Toast	370
Nine Grain	290
Plain	290
Sesame Seed	300
Chocolate Chip	360
Chocolate Raspberry	350
Choc-O-Nut	310
Cranberry Walnut	350
Morning Glory	380
P.B. Banana Crunch	390
Pumpkin	280
Spinach Parmesan	320
Trail Mix	380
Breads (2 oz Unless Noted)	
Sourdough Roll (2.5 oz)	170
Sourdough Bread Bowl (8 oz)	540
Sourdough Baguette, Round, Loaf	130
French Roll (2.25 oz)	160
French Combo Roll (5.5 oz)	340
French Loaf, Extra Large Loaf	130
French Baguette	140
Asiago Cheese Demi Loaf	150
Braided Challah	160

PANERA BREAD

Three Seed Demi	140
Olive Demi	140
Asiago Cheese Focaccia	150
Rosemary & Onion Focaccia	140
Basil Pesto Focaccia	150
Rye Loaf	140
Nine Grain	150
Honey Wheat	140
Sunflower Loaf	160
Ciabatta (6 oz)	430
Tomato Basil Extra Large Loaf	130
Cinnamon Raisin Loaf	160
Holiday Bread	150
Country Demi, Loaf, Miche	120
French Baguette, Miche	120
Multigrain Loaf, Miche	130
Sesame Semolina Demi, Loaf, Miche	130
Three Cheese Demi, Loaf, Miche	130
Stone Milled Rye Loaf, Miche	190
Kalamata Olive Demi, Loaf	140
Raisin Pecan Boule	140

Sandwiches

Turkey On Sourdough	450
Turkey On Country	590
Chicken Salad On Nine Grain	600
Chicken Salad On Sesame Semolina	690
Tuna Salad On Honey Wheat	730
Tuna Salad On Multigrain	840
Ham & Swiss On Rye	630
Ham & Swiss On Stone Milled Rye	910
PB&J On French	440
PB&J On Artisan French	560
Italian Combo On French Combo Roll	1090
Italian Combo On French Baguette	890
Italian Combo On Ciabatta	1000
Tuscan Chicken	860
Asiago Roast Beef	960
Bacon Turkey Bravo	860
Sierra Turkey	760
Garden Veggie	570
Turkey Fresco	580
Festiago Chicken On Asiago Demi	700
Turkey Artichoke	850
Frontega Chicken	860
Coronado Carnitas Panini	720

Soups (8 oz)

Black Bean	180
Boston Clam Chowder	210
Broccoli Cheddar	220
Chicken Noodle	110

PANERA BREAD

Cream of Chicken & Wild Rice	210
Garden Vegetable	100
Baked Potato	240
French Onion w/Fetina Cheese (10 oz)	200
Chicken Chili	180
Ginger Tomato Florentine	80
Moroccan Tomato Lentil	110
Potato Cream Cheese	190
Smoked Salmon & Asparagus	240
Lentil	120
Gumbo	110
Tomato Bisque	160
Forest Mushroom	140
Sante Fe Roasted Corn	140
Corn & Green Chile Chowder	190
Creamy Country Asparagus	180
Farmers' Market Bisque	140
Asiago Cheese Bisque	230
Fire Roasted Vegetable Bisque	180
Mesa Bean & Vegetable	100
Savory Vegetable Bean	120
Vegetable & Sirloin	100
Tomato Mushroom & Barley	110

Salads

Grilled Chicken Caesar	490
Caesar	390
Classic Café	400
Fandango	400
Greek	480
Asian Sesame Chicken	400
Strawberry Poppyseed	240
Tomato & Mozzarella w/Focaccia wedges	880

Spreads (2 oz)

Plain Cream Cheese	190
Average All Reduced Fat Cream Cheese	135
Roasted Garlic Hummus	90

Muffins

Banana Nut	540
Banana Nut Muffie	290
Blueberry	450
Chocolate Chip	560
Chocolate Chip Muffie	270
Pumpkin	550
Pumpkin Muffie	270
Low Fat Triple Berry	320

Danish

Apple	410
Cheese	520
Cherry	440
German Chocolate	580

Gooey Butter	600
Peach	450
Coffee Cake-Cherry Cheese	190
Croissants	
Apple	340
Butter	310
Cheese	360
Chocolate	450
Raspberry Cheese	320
Specialty Sweets	
Bear Claw	460
Cinnamon Roll	630
Cobblestone	530
Cherry Strudel	430
Apple Raisin Strudel	480
Pecan Roll	540
Cookie, Chocolate Duet w/walnuts	380
Cookie, Chocolate Chipper	410
Cookie, Nutty Oatmeal Raisin	370
Cookie, Nutty Chocolate Chipper	440
Cookie, Shortbread	390
Scone, Orange	460
Scone, Cinnamon Chip	560
Brownie, Caramel Pecan	530
Brownie, Chocolate Cream Cheese	470
Brownie, Very Chocolate	410
Bundt Cake, Carrot Walnut	590
Bundt Cake, Lemon Poppy Seed	480
Bundt Cake, Pineapple Upside-down	470
Cinnamon Almond Crunch	210

Papa John's Pizza

Original Crust Pizza (1 Slice of 14" Pizza)	Calories
Cheese	285
Chicken Alfredo	300
Garden Special	280
Meat	390
Pepperoni	305
Sausage	320
Six Cheese	425
Spinach Alfredo	335
The Works	340
Thin Crust Pizza (1 Slice of 14" Pizza)	
Cheese	235
Chicken Alfredo	270
Garden Special	225
Meat	395
Pepperoni	265
Sausage	285
Six Cheese	375

PAPA JOHN'S – PHILLY CONNECTION

Spinach Alfredo	295
The Works	320
Side Items	
BBQ	50
Bread Sticks	140
Buffalo	25
Cheese Sauce	60
Cheese Sticks	180
Chicken Strips	85
Cinnapie	115
Garlic Sauce	235
Honey Mustard	190
Pizza Sauce	25
Ranch Dressing	140

Perkins

Reduced Fat Muffins	Calories
Plain	490
Honey Bran	425
Blueberry	425
Banana	520
Reduced Fat Pies (1/6 pie)	
Wildberry	390
Apple	375
Low Fat Brownie	160
No Sugar Added Blueberry Muffin	425
Muffins	
Apple	550
Banana Nut	650
Blueberry	550
Bran	550
Carrot	455
Chocolate Chip	620
Cranberry Nut	585
Oat Bran	455
Peaches & Cream	520
Lemon Poppy seed	685
Pumpkin	550
Raspberry & Cream	585

Philly Connection

Sandwiches (Regular Size)	Calories
Cheesesteak, Original	460
Cheesesteak, Mushroom	460
Cheesesteak, Hoagie	490
Pizza Steak	470
Works	490
Steak	350
Chicken w/cheese	400

PHILLY CONNECTION – PIZZA HUT

Chicken Hoagie	430
Chicken Parmesan	440
Chicken Tenders	600
Chicken Works	440
Turkey Hoagie	420
Meatball Parmesan	590
Italian Hoagie	500
Tuna Hoagie	580
Veggie Delite Hoagie	410
Lite, Grilled Chicken	290
Lite, Chicken Hoagie	290
Lite, Turkey Hoagie	280
Lite, Veggie Hoagie	260
Lite, Chicken Parmesan	330
Lite, Chicken Works	330

Sandwiches (Large Size)

Cheesesteak, Original	710
Cheesesteak, Mushroom	720
Cheesesteak, Hoagie	750
Pizza Steak	700
Works	770
Steak	550
Chicken w/Cheese	590
Chicken Hoagie	620
Chicken Parmesan	620
Chicken Works	680
Turkey Hoagie	620
Meatball Parmesan	900
Italian Hoagie	780
Tuna Hoagie	830
Veggie Delite Hoagie	600

Salads

Veggie Delite	220
Cheesesteak	320
Chicken Tenders	340
Grilled Chicken	140
Turkey	130
Tuna	290
Garden	40
Lite, Grilled Chicken	140
Lite, Turkey	130

Pizza Hut

P'Zone (1/2)	**Calories**
Pepperoni	630
Classic	640
Meat Lover's	720
Hand Tossed Pizza (1 slice)	
Cheese	240
Beef	330

PIZZA HUT

Ham	260
Pepperoni	280
Italian Sausage	340
Pork Topping	320
Meat Lover's	320
Veggie Lover's	220
Pepperoni Lover's	250
Supreme	270
Super Supreme	290
Chicken Supreme	230

Thin'n'Crispy Pizza (1 slice)

Cheese	200
Beef	270
Ham	170
Pepperoni	190
Italian Sausage	290
Pork Topping	270
Meat Lover's	310
Veggie Lover's	190
Pepperoni Lover's	250
Supreme	250
Super Supreme	280
Chicken Supreme	200

Pan Pizza (1 Slice)

Cheese	290
Beef	330
Ham	260
Pepperoni	280
Italian Sausage	340
Pork Topping	320
Meat Lover's	360
Veggie Lover's	270
Pepperoni Lover's	330
Supreme	320
Super Supreme	340
Chicken Supreme	270

Personal Pan Pizza (1 Pizza)

Cheese	630
Ham	580
Pepperoni	620
Italian Sausage	740
Pork Topping	700
Beef Topping	710

Stuffed Crust Pizza (1 slice)

Cheese	360
Beef	390
Ham	330
Pepperoni	360
Italian Sausage	400
Pork Topping	380

Meat Lover's	470
Veggie Lover's	340
Pepperoni Lover's	420
Supreme	410
Super Supreme	430
Chicken Supreme	350

Chicago Dish Pizza (1 Slice)

Pepperoni	390
Pepperoni, Italian Sausage, Mushrooms	410
Supreme	420
Meat Lover's	470
Veggie Lover's	370

Big New Yorker Pizza (1 slice)

Cheese	410
Pepperoni	390
Ham	370
Beef Topping	500
Pork Topping	490
Italian Sausage	530
Supreme	470
Veggie Lover's	480

Stuffed Crust Gold (1 slice)

Cheese	440
Beef	490
Ham	410
Pepperoni	430
Italian Sausage	520
Pork Topping	500
Meat Lover's	550
Veggie Lover's	420
Pepperoni Lover's	500
Supreme	490
Super Supreme	510
Chicken Supreme	430
Diced Chicken	440
Sausage Lover's	520

Appetizers

Mild Buffalo Wings (5)	200
Hot Buffalo Wings (4)	210
Garlic Bread (1 Slice)	150
Breadstick (1)	130
Breadstick Dipping Sauce	30

Pasta (1 serving)

Spaghetti w/marinara	490
Spaghetti w/meat sauce	600
Spaghetti w/meatballs	850
Cavatini	480
Cavatini Supreme	560

Sandwiches

Ham & Cheese	550

Supreme	640
Desserts	
Cinnamon Sticks (2)	170
Apple Or Cherry Pizza (1 slice)	250
White Icing Dipping Cup (2 oz)	190

Qdoba

Shells	Calories
Flour Tortilla	320
Hard Taco	70
Soft Taco	95
Taco Salad	335
Tortilla Chips (Nachos)	635
Sides	
Tortilla Soup	80
Rice	200
Beans, Black Or Pinto	130
Cheese	210
Sour Cream	95
Non-fat Sour Cream	55
Guacamole	270
Fajita Vegetables	45
Meats	
Chicken	190
Steak	205
Ground Sirloin	205
Shredded Beef	215
Grilled Vegetables	50
Sauces	
Ranchero	15
Poblano Pesto	65
Mole	60
Queso	215
Corn Bean	60
Picante Ranch Dressing	175

Quizno's

Sandwiches	Calories
Small Smoked Turkey w/Raspberry Chipotle Sauce	350
Small Honey Bourbon Chicken	360
Small Turkey Lite	335

Rita's Ice

Item	Calories
Italian Ice, Kids	175
Italian Ice, Regular	275
Italian Ice, Large	435
Italian Ice, Quart	740
Sugar Free	60

RITA'S ICE – SBARRO

Cream Ice, Kids	205
Cream Ice, Regular	330
Cream Ice, Large	520
Cream Ice, Quart	880
Gelati, Regular	320
Gelati, Large	545
Gelati, Regular w/Cream Ice	345
Gelati, Large w/Cream Ice	590
Misto, Regular	415
Misto, Large	620
Misto, Regular w/Cream Ice	465
Misto, Large w/Cream Ice	695
Custard, Kids	275
Custard, Regular	370
Custard, Large	535

Ryan's

Item	Calories
Breaded Shrimp	210
Cheese Pizza (1 slice)	60
Chicken Pot Pie	150
Chicken Tenders (3)	220
Clam Chowder (1 cup)	50
Mac & Cheese (1 cup)	340
Mashed Potatoes	40
Yeast Roll	50

Sbarro

Item (1 slice or serving)	Calories
Baked Ziti	930
Cheese Calzone	775
Chicken Cutlet Parmigiana	365
Chicken Francese	390
Garlic Roll	180
Meat Lasagna	825
Mixed Vegetables	170
Pizza, Cheese	485
Pizza, Gourmet Vegetable	840
Pizza, Pepperoni	590
Pizza, Sausage	640
Pizza, Supreme	600
Salad, Caesar	395
Salad, Green Garden	50
Salad, Pasta Primavera	665
Spaghetti w/Sauce	910
Spaghetti w/Sauce & Meatballs	1310
Stuffed Pizza w/Sausage & Pepperoni	960
Stuffed Pizza w/Spinach & Broccoli	825

Schlotzsky's

Sandwiches	Calories
The Original (Sm.)	525
The Original (Reg.)	740
Large Original (Family-size)	1390
Deluxe Original (Sm.)	695
Deluxe Original (Reg.)	930
Deluxe Original (Lg.)	1785
Ham & Cheese Original (Sm.)	510
Ham & Cheese Original (Reg.)	750
Ham & Cheese Original (Lg.)	1425
Turkey Original (Sm.)	585
Turkey Original (Reg.)	820
Turkey Original (Lg.)	1570
Chicken Breast (Sm.)	340
Chicken Breast (Reg.)	500
Chicken Breast (Lg.)	980
Smoked Turkey Breast (Sm.)	335
Smoked Turkey Breast (Reg.)	500
Smoked Turkey Breast (Lg.)	990
The Vegetarian (Sm.)	325
The Vegetarian (Reg.)	480
The Vegetarian (Lg.)	935
Albacore Tuna (Sm.)	335
Albacore Tuna (Reg.)	495
Albacore Tuna (Lg.)	970
Fiesta Chicken (Sm.)	580
Fiesta Chicken (Reg.)	840
Fiesta Chicken (Lg.)	1600
Roast Beef & Cheese (Sm.)	585
Roast Beef & Cheese (Reg.)	855
Roast Beef & Cheese (Lg.)	1640
Turkey & Bacon Club (Sm.)	570
Turkey & Bacon Club (Reg.)	835
Turkey & Bacon Club (Lg.)	1590
Pastrami & Swiss (Sm.)	585
Pastrami & Swiss (Reg.)	880
Pastrami & Swiss (Lg.)	1750
Hot Sandwiches, Limited Time Offer	
Albuquerque Turkey (Sm.)	635
Albuquerque Turkey (Reg.)	920
Albuquerque Turkey (Lg.)	1650
All American Angus (Sm.)	630
All American Angus (Reg.)	900
All American Angus (Lg.)	1710
Hot Sandwiches, Where Available	
Dijon Chicken (Sm.)	330
Dijon Chicken (Reg.)	495
Dijon Chicken (Lg.)	970

SCHLOTZSKY'S

Santa Fe Chicken (Sm.)	405
Santa Fe Chicken (Reg.)	605
Santa Fe Chicken (Lg.)	1150
Pesto Chicken (Sm.)	345
Pesto Chicken (Reg.)	510
Pesto Chicken (Lg.)	1000
Chicken Club (Sm.)	460
Chicken Club (Reg.)	685
Chicken Club (Lg.)	1350
The Philly (Sm.)	570
The Philly (Reg.)	840
The Philly (Lg.)	1615
Corned Beef Rueben (Sm.)	535
Corned Beef Rueben (Reg.)	840
Corned Beef Rueben (Lg.)	1630
Corned Beef (Sm.)	395
Corned Beef (Reg.)	595
Corned Beef (Lg.)	1170
Pastrami Rueben (Sm.)	635
Pastrami Rueben (Reg.)	945
Pastrami Rueben (Lg.)	1845
Roast Beef (Sm.)	420
Roast Beef (Reg.)	625
Roast Beef (Lg.)	1220
Turkey Rueben (Sm.)	555
Turkey Rueben (Reg.)	825
Turkey Rueben (Lg.)	1600
Albacore Tuna Melt (Sm.)	510
Albacore Tuna Melt (Reg.)	740
Albacore Tuna Melt (Lg.)	1400
Western Vegetarian (Sm.)	425
Western Vegetarian (Reg.)	610
Western Vegetarian (Lg.)	1205
Vegetable Club (Sm.)	370
Vegetable Club (Reg.)	540
Vegetable Club (Lg.)	1055
BLT (Sm.)	380
BLT (Reg.)	580
BLT (Lg.)	1140
Turkey Guacamole (Sm.)	425
Turkey Guacamole (Reg.)	645
Turkey Guacamole (Lg.)	1260
Texas Schlotzsky's® (Sm.)	540
Texas Schlotzsky's® (Reg.)	775
Texas Schlotzsky's® (Lg.)	1490
Pizza, 8"	
Double Cheese & Pepperoni	720
Barbeque Chicken	685
Vegetarian Special	550
Thai Chicken	665

SCHLOTZSKY'S

The Original Combination	625
Tuscan Herb	540
Three Meat	805
Kung Pao Chicken	720
Kid's Cheese	460
Kid's Pepperoni	505
Chicken & Pesto	650
Smoked Turkey & Jalapeño	625
Double Cheese	580
Bacon, Tomato & Mushroom	610
Fresh Tomato & Pesto	540
Mediterranean	525

Wraps

Asian Almond Chicken	460
Salsa Chicken w/Cheddar	460
Zesty Albacore Tuna	310
Chicken Caesar	510

Deli Salads

Fresh Fruit Salad	125
Fresh Fruit Salad (Sm.)	85
Chicken & Pesto Pasta Salad	455
Chicken & Pesto Pasta Salad (Sm.)	325
Chicken Salad	375
Chicken Salad (Sm.)	285
Albacore Tuna Salad	220
Albacore Tuna Salad (Sm.)	135
Potato Salad	290
Mustard Potato Salad	250
Homestyle Cole Slaw	190
Elbow Macaroni Salad	275
California Pasta Salad	60
Chicken Caesar	110
Caesar	30
Smoked Turkey Chef's	200
Garden	50
Small Garden	25
Chinese Chicken	130
Greek	160
Ham & Turkey Chef's	200

Salad Dressings & Extras

Traditional Ranch	270
Spicy Ranch	230
Light Spicy Ranch	140
Light Italian	90
Thousand Island	220
Olde World Caesar	260
Greek Balsamic Vinaigrette	170
Sesame Ginger Vinaigrette	170
Chow Mien Noodles	75
Garlic Cheese Croutons	45

SCHLOTZSKY'S – SHONEY'S

Chips

Barbeque	210
Jalapeño	210
Regular (Plain)	210
Salt & Vinegar	210
Sour Cream & Onion	210
Cracked Pepper	210

Kids Deals

Cheese Pizza	460
Cheese Sandwich	400
PBJ Sandwich	470
Ham & Cheese Sandwich	430
Pepperoni Pizza	505

Desserts

Chocolate Chip Cookie	160
Oatmeal Raisin Cookie	150
Peanut Butter Cookie	170
Sugar Cookie	160
White Chocolate Macadamia Cookie	170
Fudge Chocolate Chip Cookie	170
New York Creamstyle Cheesecake	310
Strawberry Swirl Cheesecake	300
Cookies & Creme Cheesecake	330
Fudge Brownie Cake	410
Cranberry Walnut Crunch	160
Golden Raisin Oatmeal	160
Triple Chocolate Chip	170
Cookies w/Real M&M's®	140

Bread

Sourdough Bun (Sm.)	225
Sourdough Bun (Reg.)	335
Sourdough Bun (Lg.)	670
Wheat Bun (Sm.)	225
Wheat Bun (Reg.)	335
Dark Rye Bun (Sm.)	220
Dark Rye Bun (Reg.)	330
Jalapeño Cheese Bun (Sm.)	235
Jalapeño Cheese Bun (Reg.)	355
Pizza Crust	330

Shoney's

Blue Plate Specials	Calories
Baked Whitefish	505
Cajun Whitefish	480
Grandma's Meat Loaf – w/glaze	1090
Grandma's Meat Loaf – w/gravy	1090
Grilled Liver 'n' Onions	710
Ham Steak Dinner	670
Original Country Fried Steak	1150
Roast Beef Platter	880

SHONEY'S

Sides/Condiments

Mashed Potatoes/Gravy	220
Corn	175
Green Beans	125
Macaroni & Cheese	240
Bread Service – 2 Sl. w/Oleo	265
Cranberry Sauce, 1.5 ox.	65

Breakfast Menu Selections

All Star Breakfast (Add Options)	190
BigEater Steak Breakfast (Add Options)	630
Country Fried Steak Breakfast	995
Deluxe Pancake Platter	1610
Half Stack Pancake Platter	930
Sausage/Biscuit [1]	540
Sunrise Breakfast	970

Breakfast Sides

Bacon (3 strips)	120
Biscuits & Gravy	685
Sausage Patties (each)	210
Hashbrowns – 4 oz	240
Grits – 4 oz	105
Biscuits (each)	310
White Toast – 2 sl. w/margarine	200
Wheat Toast – 2 sl. w/margarine	190
Sourdough Toast – 2 sl. w/margarine	205
Apple Cinnamon Jelly – 1 pack	35
Grape Jelly – 1 pack	35
Strawberry Jam – 1 pack	35
Margarine – 1 pack (5 g)	35
Creamer, Half & Half® – 1 container (15 g)	20

Breakfast Bar

Bacon – 3 strips	120
Banana – 7"– 8" Long (118 g)	110
Biscuit (each)	310
Blackberries, 1/4 Cup (36 g)	20
Blueberries, 1/4 Cup (36.3 g)	20
Breakfast Bar Gravy – 2 oz	55
Breakfast Potato Casserole – 4 oz	40
Cake, Brunch Berry	120

Cake, Bundt Variety (each)

Apple Spice	120
Banana Bash	130
Buttercreme	130
Double Chocolate	130
Luscious Lemon	130
Orange Cranberry	120

Various

Cottage Cheese – 1 Tblsp (16.4 g)	15
DoNuts, Powdered – each (35.4 g)	175
Eggs, Breakfast Bar – 1/2 cup (128 g)	120

SHONEY'S

French Toast Sticks – 4 pieces (98 g)	380
Grits – 4 oz.	105
Ham, Diced – 1 Tblsp (9.1 g)	15
Hashbrowns – 4 oz	240
Honey, Individual – 1 Pack	45
Jelly, Apple/Cinnamon – 1 Pack	35
Jelly, Grape – 1 Pack	35
Jelly, Strawberry Jam – 1 Pack	35
Milk, White – 1/2 Cup (122 g)	75
Oleo Margarine, Country Crock Individuals	35
Omelet Topping – 1 oz	20
Pancakes (each)	320
Salad, Tropical Fruit – 1/4 Cup (60 g)	50
Sausage Patty – Each (56.7 g)	210
Smoked Sausage, Sliced – 1 sli (56 g)	180
Strawberry Banana Topping – 4 oz	85
Syrup, Diet, Smuckers – 1 Ladle (28.4 g)	45
Syrup, Pancake & Waffle – 2 Tblsp	80
Topping, Apple – 1/4 Cup (62 g)	95
Topping, Apple Crisp – 1/4 Cup (62 g)	90
Topping, Peach – 1/4 Cup (62 g)	55
Topping, Strawberry – 1/4 Cup (62 g)	160
Tortillas, Flour – Each	135
Whipped Topping – 1 Scoop (3.6 g)	10
Burgers	
All-American Bacon Cheeseburger	890
All-American Burger	670
Famous Patty Melt	945
Half-O-Pound Burger	1350
Mushroom Swiss Burger	970
Add-Ons/Sides	
American Cheese, 1 slice	105
Bacon, per slice	40
BBQ Sauce, per 1.5 oz	70
Cocktail Sauce, per 1.5 oz.	55
French Fries (4 oz)	210
Grilled Onions – 1.5 oz	70
Monterey Jack Cheese, 1 slice	160
Onion Rings – 1 order (7 rings)	500
Sauteed Mushrooms – 3 oz	105
Secret Sauce, per 1.5 oz.	170
Sweet & Sour Sauce, per 1.5 oz	70
Swiss Cheese, 1 slice	160
Tartar Sauce, per 1.5 oz	225
Chicken	
Charbroiled Blackened Chicken	830
Charbroiled Chicken Breast	795
Chicken Stir-Fry	1200
Fried Chicken Tenderloins	1160
Monterey Chicken	910

SHONEY'S

Smothered Chicken	890
Desserts	
Apple Nutrasweet Pie	455
Apple Pie A la Mode	1205
Caramel Sundae	620
Cheesecake - 1 slice (4 oz)	365
Cherry Nutrasweet Pie	470
Chocolate Milk Shake	1085
Hot Fudge Sundae	600
Original Strawberry Pie - 1 slice	330
Peach Nutrasweet Pie	480
Strawberry Milk Shake	1115
Strawberry Sundae	610
Ultimate Hot Fudge Cake	875
Vanilla Milk Shake	1075
Walnut Brownie a la Mode	575
Drinks	
Hot Chocolate	120
Iced Tea, Sweetened (26 oz)	365
Junior Meals	
Junior Chicken	190
Junior Fish & Chips	310
Pasta	
Chicken Alfredo	1705
Italian Feast	1435
Pasta Ya Ya	1850
Shrimp Alfredo	1780
Condiments/Sides	
Bread Service - 2 slices w/margarine	265
Cheese, Parmesan - 1 Tblsp	20
Sandwiches	
Blackened Chicken Sandwich	885
Charbroiled Chicken Sandwich	895
Chicken Parmesan Sandwich	750
Corned Beef Reuben	790
Fish Sandwich	830
Fried Chicken Sandwich	560
Hot Roast Beef Sandwich w/mashed potatoes & gravy	770
Hot Turkey Sandwich w/mashed potatoes & gravy	840
Original Slim Jim	1005
Raymond's French Dip	500
Turkey Club	950
Ultimate Grilled Cheese	895
Salad	
Dave's Pasta - 2/3 cup	170
Macaroni - 1/2 Cup	310
Potato, Classic - 1/2 Cup	190
Red Potato - 1/2 Cup	280
Sweet Potato Casserole - 4 oz	245

SHONEY'S – SKYLINE CHILI

Seafood

Fried Fish Platter	1050
Grilled Cod, Lite	200
Grilled Salmon	750
Grilled Salmon, Lite	180
Grilled Shrimp	720
Grilled Shrimp, Lite	320
Shrimp Stir-Fry	875
Shrimper's Feast	1030

Seafood Bar

Cheese, Deli Spread - 1 Tblsp	70
Cheese, Parmesan - 1 Tblsp	20
Cole Slaw - 1/4 cup	125
Corn, Seasoned - 4 oz	175
Crackers, Club - 1 pack (7 g)	30
Crackers, Oyster - 10 crackers	180
Crackers, Saltines - 1 Pack (5.9 g)	25
Gravy, Brown - 2 oz	35
Macaroni & Cheese - 1/2 cup	240
Mashed Potatoes - 6 oz	1890
Okra, breaded - 4 oz	300
Margarine (individual)	35
Pinto Beans - 4 oz	135
Yeast Roll	115

Steaks

12-oz. T-Bone	1810
6-oz Choice Sirloin	1225
8-oz. Ribeye	1480
BBQ Ribs	1520
Half-O-Pound w/ Grilled. Mushrooms	1315
Half-O-Pound w/ Grilled. Onions	1335

Rib Combos (w/fries)

1/4 Rack & BBQ Chicken	1230
1/4 Rack & Tenderloins	1370
1/4 Rack & Fried Shrimp	1145
1/4 Rack & Grilled Shrimp	1125
Southwest Half-O-Pound	1305

Surf & Turf

Ribeye & 5 Fried Shrimp	1640
Ribeye & 6 Grilled Shrimp	1590
Sirloin & 5 Fried Shrimp	1380
Sirloin & 6 Grilled Shrimp	1330
T-Bone & 5 Fried Shrimp	1965
T-Bone & 6 Grilled Shrimp	1920

Skyline Chili

Item	Calories
Black Beans And Rice	330
Cheese Coney	350

SKYLINE CHILI – SMOOTHIE KING

Cheese SkyFries	660
Chili Cheese SkyFries	810
Chili Sandwich	190
Chili Sandwich w/cheese	300
Deluxe Burrito	640
Kid-Sized SkyFries	210
Large 3-Way	1050
Large 4-Way	1070
Large 4-Way w/Beans	1160
Large 5-Way	1180
Large Chili Spaghetti	540
Large Chili Spaghetti Beans & Onions	660
Large Chili Spaghetti w/Beans	650
Large Chili Spaghetti w/Onions	550
Large Garden Salad	150
Large Greek Salad	690
Large Nacho Salad	750
Regular 3-Way	710
Regular 4-Way	720
Regular 4-Way w/Beans	780
Regular 5-Way	790
Regular Burrito	570
Regular Chili Plain	250
Regular Chili Plain w/Beans	260
Regular Chili Spaghetti	400
Regular Chili Spaghetti Beans & Onions	490
Regular Chili Spaghetti w/Beans	480
Regular Chili Spaghetti w/Onions	410
Regular Coney	240
Regular Garden Salad	80
Regular Greek Salad	370
Regular Nacho Salad	450
SkyFries	430

Smoothie King

Smoothies	Calories
Activator, Chocolate	430
Activator, Vanilla	430
Activator, Strawberry	560
Almond Mocha	400
Angel Food	330
Banana	410
Banana Boat	520
Blackberry Dream	345
Blueberry Heaven	260
Caribbean Way	390
Celestial Cherry High	285
Cherry Picker	360
Chocolate	400
Coconut Surprise	460

SMOOTHIE KING

Cranberry Cooler	540
Cranberry Supreme	580
Grape Expectations	400
Grape Expectations II	530
Hearty Apple	380
Hulk, Chocolate	845
Hulk, Strawberry	955
Hulk, Vanilla	745
Immune Builder	335
Instant Vigor	360
Island Treat	335
Lemon	390
Lemon Twist Banana	340
Lemon Twist Strawberry	400
Light & Fluffy	390
Malts	890
Mangofest	320
Mo'cuccino	420
Muscle Punch Plus	340
Muscle Punch Plus	340
Orange Ka-bam	320
Peach Slice Plus	470
Peach Slice Plus	340
Peanut Power	500
Peanut Power Plus, Grape	705
Peanut Power Plus, Strawberry	630
Pep Upper	335
Pina Colada Island	550
Pineapple	380
Pineapple Pleaser	315
Pineapple Surf	440
Power Punch	430
Power Punch Plus	500
Raspberry Sunrise	335
Shakes	875
Slim-n-trim Chocolate	270
Slim-n-trim Orange Vanilla	200
Slim-n-trim Strawberry	360
Slim-n-trim Vanilla	230
Strawberry Kiwi Breeze	300
Strawberry X-treme	370
Super power punch	515
Super punch	425
Yogurt D-Lite	335
Youth Fountain	370
Kids' Kup Smoothies	
Berry Interesting	150
Choc-A-Laka	210
Gimme-Grape	170
Smarti Tarti	150

SouperSalad

Dressing	Calories
Blue Cheese	130
Fat-free Cranberry Vinaigrette	10
Fat-free French Dressing	30
Fat-free Italian w/cheese	15
French Dijon Mustard	10
Gourmet Mayonnaise	100
Greek Dressing	100
Green Goddess	130
Honey Mustard	120
Hot Bacon	140
House Vinaigrette	110
Tableside Caesar	140
Tangy Oriental	70
Thousand Island	150

Soup	
Beef Stroganoff	350
Chicken Creole	320
Chicken Tetrazini	350
Cream of Cauliflower	190
Cream of Mushroom	225
Cream of Spinach	80
German Potato	320
Hungarian Mushroom	350
Mac and Cheese	350
Mama Mia Chicken	320
New England Clam Chowder	290
Potato Leek	255
Santa Fe Chicken	320
Shrimp Creole	255
Tomato Basil	225
Mexican Corn Chowder	225
Mushroom Cheese Soup	255
Potato Corn Chowder	320

Bread	
Blueberry Bread	260
Cornbread	60
Focaccia Bread	390
Garlic Bread Stick	120
GingerBread	290
Jalapeno Cheddar Focaccia	70
Mediterranean Focaccia	70

Steak Escape

7" Sandwiches	Calories
Great Escape	510
Grand Escape	515

STEAK ESCAPE

Wild West BBQ	550
Turkey Club	500
Grand Gobbler	510
Grandest Chicken	510
Ragin' Cajun	520
Hambrosia	490
Vegetarian	500
12" Sandwiches	
Great Escape	840
Grand Escape	840
Wild West BBQ	920
Turkey Club	765
Grand Gobbler	740
Grandest Chicken	830
Ragin' Cajun	815
Hambrosia	730
Vegetarian	690
Kids Sandwiches	
Steak & Cheese	260
Chicken & Cheese	255
Turkey & Cheese	235
Ham & Cheese	235
All White Meat Tenders (2)	240
Smashed Potatoes	
Plain	370
w/Steak	540
w/Chicken	530
w/Turkey	485
w/Ham	485
Loaded Smashed Potatoes	
Bacon & Cheddar	635
Ranch & Bacon	690
Fresh Salads	
Side Salad	190
Grilled Salad w/steak	340
Grilled Salad w/chicken	330
Grilled Salad w/turkey	285
Grilled Salad w/ham	285
Fresh-Cut French Fries	
Kids Meal Fries	250
12 oz cup	500
16 oz cup	650
25 oz cup	920
32 oz cup	995
Loaded French Fries	
Bacon & Cheddar	905
Ranch & Bacon	1045
Toppings	
Provolone Cheese	105
Swiss Cheese	100

STEAK ESCAPE – SUBWAY

Cheddar Cheese	115
American Cheese-White	100
Mayonnaise	100
Brown Mustard	0
BBQ Sauce	40
Italian Dressing	50
Ranch Dressing	85
Margarine	205
Sour Cream	60
Lettuce	0
Tomato	25
Mild Peppers	10
Jalapeno Peppers	10
Black Olives	30
Bacon	80
Fresh-Squeezed Lemonade	
12 oz	125
16 oz	170
21 oz	235
32 oz	340
44 oz	490

Subway

Sandwiches	Calories
6" Cold Cut Trio™	440
6" Ham	290
6" Italian BMT®	480
6" Meatball	540
6" Roast Beef	290
6" Roasted Chicken Breast	320
6" Steak & Cheese	390
6" Subway Club®	320
6" Subway Melt®	410
6" Subway Seafood & Crab®	410
6" Tuna	450
6" Turkey Breast	280
6" Turkey Breast & Ham	290
6" Veggie Delite®	230
Barbecue Pulled Pork	440
BBQ Rib Patty	420
Buffalo Chicken	400
Chicken Pizziola	460
Chipotle Southwest Steak&Cheese	440
Chipotle Southwest Turkey Bacon	410
Dijon Horseradish Melt	470
Double Meat Chicken	410
Double Meat Cold Cut Trio™	580
Double Meat Ham	350
Double Meat Italian BMT®	670

SUBWAY

Double Meat Meatball	780
Double Meat Roast Beef	360
Double Meat Steak & Cheese	480
Double Meat Subway Club®	410
Double Meat Subway Melt®	520
Double Meat Subway Seafood & Crab®	510
Double Meat Tuna	590
Double Meat Turkey Breast	340
Double Meat Turkey Breast & Ham	360
Extreme Dijon Horseradish Melt	540
Extreme Red Wine Vinaigrette Club	450
Extreme Southwest Turkey Bacon	470
Extreme Sweet Onion Chicken Teriyaki	450
Gardenburger®	390
Ham On Deli Round	210
Honey Mustard Ham	310
Lloyd's BBQ Chicken	330
Mediterranean Chicken	470
Pastrami	570
Pizza Sub	460
Red Wine Vinaigrette Club	350
Roast Beef On Deli Round	220
Spicy Italian	480
Sweet Onion Chicken Teriyaki	380
Thai Sesame Chicken	370
Tuna On Deli Round	330
Turkey Breast On Deli Round	220
Veggie-Max	390

Salads

Cold Cut Trio™	230
Ham	110
Italian BMT®	280
Meatball	330
Roast Beef	120
Roasted Chicken Breast	140
Seafood & Crab®	200
Steak & Cheese	180
Subway Club®	150
Subway Melt®	200
Tuna	240
Turkey Breast	100
Turkey Breast & Ham	120
Veggie Delite®	50

Breakfast Sandwich On Deli Round

Bacon & Egg	320
Cheese & Egg	320
Ham & Egg	310
Steak & Egg	330
Vegetable & Egg	290
Western & Egg	300

SUBWAY

Breakfast Sandwich On 6" Italian Or Wheat Bread

Bacon & Egg	450
Cheese & Egg	440
Ham & Egg	430
Steak & Egg	460
Vegetable & Egg	410
Western & Egg	430

Omelets & French Toast

Bacon & Egg (1)	240
Cheese & Egg	240
French Toast w/ Syrup	350
Ham & Egg	230
Steak & Egg	250
Vegetable & Egg	210
Western & Egg	220

Cookies & Desserts

Apple Pie	245
Chocolate Chip Cookie	220
Chocolate Chunk Cookie	220
Double Chocolate Chip Cookie	210
M & M® Cookie	220
Oatmeal Raisin Cookie	200
Peanut Butter Cookie	220
Sugar Cookie	230
White Macadamia Nut Cookie	220

Soup (1 cup)

Black Bean	180
Brown And Wild Rice w/Chicken	190
Cheese w/Ham And Bacon	230
Chicken And Dumpling	130
Chili Con Carne	310
Cream of Broccoli	130
Cream of Potato w/Bacon	210
Golden Broccoli Cheese	480
Minestrone	70
New England Style Clam Chowder	140
Potato Cheese Chowder	210
Roasted Chicken Noodle	90
Tomato Bisque	90
Vegetable Beef	90

Breads

6" Hearty Italian	210
6" Honey Oat	250
6" Italian (white)	200
6" Italian Herbs & Cheese	240
6" Monterey Cheddar	240
6" Parmesan Oregano	210
6" Roasted Garlic	230
6" Sourdough	210
6" Wheat	200

SUBWAY – SWEET TOMATOES

Deli Style Roll	170
Wrap	200
Sides, Sauces & Condiments	
Bacon (2 Strips)	45
Chipotle Southwest	90
Dijon Horseradish	90
Fat-Free French	70
Fat-Free Honey Mustard	30
Fat-Free Italian	20
Fat-Free Ranch	60
Fat-Free Red Wine Vinaigrette	30
Fat-Free Sweet Onion	40
Meats (Amount On 6" sub)	
Cold Cut Trio™ Meats	140
Ham	60
Italian BMT® Meats	180
Meatball	240
Roast Beef	70
Roasted Chicken	90
Steak (no cheese)	90
Subway Club® Meats	100
Subway Seafood & Crab®	110
Tuna	150
Turkey Breast	50

Sweet Tomatoes & Souplantation

Tossed Salads (1 Cup)	Calories
Bartlett Pear & Walnut Salad	180
BBQ Julienne Chopped Salad	190
Caesar Salad Asiago	190
California Cobb Salad	180
Cape Cod Spinach w/walnuts	170
Chicken Tortilla Salad	180
Classic Antipasto Salad w/peppered salami	140
Country French Salad w/bacon	210
Ensalada Azteca Salad	130
Greek Salad	120
Italian Sub Salad w/turkey & salami	260
Mandarin Spinach Salad w/caramelized walnuts	170
Mediterranean Salad	150
Monterey Blue Salad w/peanuts	200
Pesto Orzo Salad w/pinenuts	220
Ragin' Cajun Salad	200
Ranch House BLT Salad w/turkey	180
Roasted Vegetables Salad w/feta cheese & olives	140
Roma Tomato, Mozzarella & Basil Salad	120
Smoked Turkey & Spinach Salad w/almonds	190
Sonoma Spinach Salad w/Honey Dijon Vinaigrette	210
Spiced Pecan & Roasted Vegetable	180

SWEET TOMATOES & SOUPLANTATION

Spinach Gorgonzola w/spiced pecans	210
Strawberry Fields w/caramelized walnuts	130
Summer Lemon w/spiced pecans	220
Traditional Spinach Salad w/bacon	160
Watercress & Orange Salad	90
Won Ton Chicken Happiness	150

Salads (1/2 Cup)

Ambrosia w/Coconut	170
Artichoke Rice Salad	160
Aunt Doris' Red Pepper Slaw (Fat-Free)	70
Baja Bean & Cilantro Salad (Low-Fat)	180
BBQ Potato Salad	160
Carrot Ginger Salad w/Herb Vinaigrette	150
Carrot Raisin Salad (low fat)	90
Chinese Krab Salad	160
Citrus Noodles Salad w/snow peas	140
Dijon Potato Salad w/Garlic Dill Vinaigrette	150
German Potato Salad (low-fat)	120
Greek Couscous Salad w/feta cheese	170
Italian Garden Vegetable Salad	110
Italian White Bean Salad	140
Jalapeno Potato Salad	140
Joan's Broccoli Madness Salad	180
Lemon Rice w/cashews	160
Mandarin Noodles Salad w/ broccoli (low-fat)	120
Mandarin Shells Salad w/almonds	120
Marinated Summer Vegetables Salad (fat-free)	80
Moroccan Marinated Vegetables Salad (low-fat)	90
Old Fashioned Macaroni Salad w/ham	180
Oriental Ginger Slaw w/Krab (low-fat)	70
Penne Pasta Salad w/Chicken in Citrus Vinigarette (low-fat)	130
Pesto Pasta Salad	160
Picnic Potato Salad	150
Pineapple Coconut Slaw	150
Poppyseed Coleslaw	120
Red Potato & Tomato	120
Roasted Potato Salad w/Chipotle Chile Vinaigrette	140
Shrimp & Seafood Shells Salad	200
Southern Dill Potato Salad (low-fat)	120
Southwestern Rice & Beans Salad	90
Spicy Southwestern Pasta Salad (low-fat)	130
Summer Barley Salad w/Black Beans (low-fat)	110
Thai Noodle Salad w/peanut sauce	170
Three Bean Marinade Salad	170
Tomato Cucumber Marinade Salad	80
Tuna Tarragon Salad	240
Turkey Chutney Pasta Salad	230
Wild Rice & Chicken Salad	300
Zesty Tortellini Salad	190

SWEET TOMATOES & SOUPLANTATION

Dressings (2 Tblsp)

Bacon	120
Balsamic Vinaigrette	180
Basil Vinaigrette	160
Blue Cheese	140
Creamy Italian	120
Cucumber (reduced-calorie)	80
fat-free Honey Mustard (fat-free)	45
fat-free Italian (fat-free)	20
fat-free Ranch (fat-free)	50
Honey Mustard	150
Kahlena French	120
Parmesan Pepper Cream	160
Ranch	130
Roasted Garlic	140
Thousand Island	110
Croutons, Garlic Parmesan Seasoned (low-fat, 5 pieces)	40
Croutons, Tomato Basil (5 pieces)	45

Soup (1 cup)

Albino Bean Chicken Cuisine	190
Albondigas Buenas (meatball soup)	190
Arizona Chili	220
Baked Potato & Cheese w/bacon	290
Be Wild w/Mushroom	220
Big Chunk Chicken Noodle (low-fat)	160
Black Bean Sausage Fling	350
Broc On	220
Butternut Squash Soup (vegetarian)	140
Cheatin' Heart Chili	300
Chesapeake Corn Chowder	310
Chicken Fajitas & Black Bean Soup	280
Chicken Got Smoked	350
Chicken Pot Pie Stew	310
Chicken Tortilla w/Jalapeno Chilis & Tomatoes (low-fat)	100
Chunky Potato Cheese Soup w/Thyme	210
Country Corn & Red Potato Chowder	160
Cream of Broccoli Soup (vegetarian)	210
Cream of Chicken Soup	250
Cream of Mushroom Soup (non-vegetarian)	290
Creamy Vegetable Chowder	200
Deep Kettle House Chili (low-fat)	230
Deep Kettle House Chili w/ 33% more meat!	250
Devotion To The Ocean	220
Do The Stew!	280
Do The Stew! w/barley	290
El Paso Lime & Chicken Soup	160
French Onion Soup (low-fat)	80
Garden Fresh Vegetable Soup (low-fat)	110

SWEET TOMATOES & SOUPLANTATION

Garlic Kickin Roasted Chicken	140
Green Chile Stew	150
Hungarian Vegetable (low-fat)	120
Irish Potato Leek Soup (vegetarian)	260
Living On The Veg	90
Lonely For Minestrone	150
Longhorn Beef Chili	190
Make Room For Mushroom	240
Manhattan Clam Chowder	130
Marvelous Minestrone Soup	210
Minestrone w/Italian Sausage	210
Mulligatawny Soup	210
Navy Bean Soup w/ham	340
Neighbor Joe's Gumbo	280
New Orleans Jambalaya	210
Not Skimpy On The Shrimpy	290
Old Fashion Vegetable Soup (low-fat/vegetarian/ no cholesterol)	100
Posole Soup	150
Potato Sprung a Leek	190
Rock N' Mole Chili	240
Santa Fe Black Bean Chili (low-fat/vegetarian)	190
Shrimp Bisque	300
Southwest Tomato Cream Soup	120
Spicy 4-Bean Minestrone (low-fat/vegetarian)	140
Spicy Sausage & Pasta Soup	310
Split Pea Soup w/ham	350
Sweet Tomato Cream Soup	180
Sweet Tomato Onion Soup (low-fat/vegetarian)	110
Texas Red Chili	240
Three-Bean Turkey Chili (low-fat/high-fiber/no dairy)	140
Tomato Parmesan & Vegetables (low-fat/vegetarian w/dairy)	120
Toot Your Horn For Crab & Corn	290
Tortellini Soup	180
Turkey Vegetable Soup	270
Tuscany Chicken Stew	190
Vegetable Beef Stew	250
Vegetable Medley Soup (low-fat/vegetarian)	90
Vegetarian Chili (vegetarian)	150
Vegetarian Harvest Soup (vegetarian)	190
Vegetarian Lentils & Brown Rice (low-fat/vegetarian)	130
Veggie Jackson	100
Very Nice Chicken & Rice	160
Yankee Clipper Clam Chowder w/bacon	330
Muffins & Breads (each)	
Apple Cinnamon Bran Muffin (96% fat-free)	80
Apple Raisin Muffin	150
Banana Nut Muffin	150
Big Blue Blueberry Muffin	310

SWEET TOMATOES & SOUPLANTATION

Big Hearth Pizza Focaccia	140
Black Forest Muffin	230
Bruschetta Focaccia	130
Buttermilk Cornbread (low-fat)	140
Cappuccino Chip Muffin	160
Caribbean Key Lime Muffin	170
Carrot Pineapple Muffin w/oat bran	150
Cherry Nut Muffin	150
Chile Corn Muffin (low-fat)	140
Chocolate Brownie Muffin	170
Chocolate Chip Muffin	170
Country Blackberry Muffin	170
Cranberry Orange Bran Muffin (96% fat-free)	80
French Quarter Praline Muffin	290
Fruit Medley Bran Muffin (96% fat-free)	80
Garlic Parmesan Focaccia (low-fat)	100
Georgia Peach Poppyseed Muffin	150
Indian Grain Bread (low-fat)	200
Lemon Muffin	140
Macadamia Nut Spice Muffin	220
Maple Walnut Muffin	230
Nutty Peanut Butter Muffin	170
Pauline's Apple Walnut Cake	180
Pepperoni Focaccia	180
Pumpkin Raisin Muffin	150
Roasted Potato Focaccia	150
Sauteed Vegetable Focaccia	150
Sourdough Bread (low-fat)	150
Strawberry Buttermilk Muffin	140
Sweet Orange & Cranberry Muffin	200
Taffy Apple Muffin	160
Tomatillo Focaccia	140
Tropical Papaya Coconut Muffin	180
Zucchini Nut Muffin	150
Pastas (1 cup)	
Beef Stroganoff	340
Broccoli Alfredo w/basil	380
Bruschetta	260
Carbonara Pasta	280
Cilantro Lime Pesto	370
Creamy Bruschetta	360
Creamy Herb Chicken	310
Creamy Pepper Jack	290
Fettuccine Alfredo	390
Garden Vegetable w/Italian sausage	300
Garden Vegetable w/meatballs	270
Greek Mediterranean	290
Italian Sausage w/red pepper puree	250
Italian Vegetable Beef	270
Lemon Cream & Asparagus	230

SWEET TOMATOES & SOUPLANTATION – TCBY

Linguini w/Clam Sauce	380
Macaroni & Cheese	260
Nutty Mushroom	390
Oriental Green Bean & Noodle (low-fat)	240
Pasta Florentine	360
Smoked Salmon & Dill	360
Southwestern Alfredo Pasta	350
Tuscany Sausage w/capers & olives	240
Vegetable Ragu	250
Vegetarian Marinara w/basil	260
Walnut Pesto	310

Desserts (1/2 Cup)

Apple Cobbler	350
Apple Medley (fat-free)	70
Banana Pudding	160
Banana Royale (fat-free)	80
Blissful Blueberry Cobbler	380
Butterscotch Praline Cake	220
Butterscotch Pudding (low-fat)	140
Candy Sprinkles - 1 Tblsp. (low-fat)	70
Cherry Cobbler	340
Chocolate Chip Cookie - 1 Small	70
Chocolate Frozen Yogurt (fat-free)	95
Chocolate Lava Cake	295
Chocolate Pudding (low-fat)	140
Chocolate Pudding (low-fat) (No Sugar Added)	90
Chocolate Syrup - 2 Tblsp. (fat-free)	70
Cranberry Apple Cobbler	370
Granola Topping - 2 Tblsp.	110
Jello (flavored) (fat-free)	80
Jello (sugar-free, flavored, fat-free)	10
Nutty Waldorf Salad (low-fat)	80
Peach Cobbler	360
Rice Pudding (low-fat)	110
Tapioca Pudding (low-fat)	140
Vanilla Pudding	140
Vanilla Soft Serve (reduced fat)	140

TCBY

Soft Serve Frozen Yogurt (1/2 cup)	Calories
Non-fat	110
Non-fat (no sugar added)	90
96% fat-free	140
Non-Fat & Non-Dairy Sorbet	100

Juice Smoothies

Mighty Berry	300
Passion Power	300
Raging Raspberry	300
Pineapple Combustion	340

TCBY - TACO BELL

Non-fat Yogurt Smoothies

Banana Berry Blast-off	400
Strawberry Surge	400
Latter Cooler	400
Raspberry Rush	340
Pina-Chillada	440
Tropical Bliss	360
Peanut Butter Fusion	730

Golden Vanilla Yogurt Smoothies

Banana Berry Blast-off	410
Strawberry Surge	410
Latter Cooler	420
Raspberry Rush	360
Pina-Chillada	450
Tropical Bliss	370
Peanut Butter Fusion	740

Taco Bell

Taco	Calories
Taco	170
Taco Supreme®	220
Soft Taco - Beef	210
Soft Taco - Chicken	190
Soft Taco Supreme® - Beef	260
Soft Taco Supreme® - Chicken	230
Grilled Steak Soft Taco	280
Double Decker® Taco	340
Double Decker® Taco Supreme®	280
Gordita	
Gordita Supreme® - Beef	310
Gordita Supreme® - Chicken	290
Gordita Supreme® - Steak	290
Gordita Baja® - Beef	350
Gordita Baja® - Chicken	320
Gordita Baja® - Steak	320
Gordita Nacho Cheese - Beef	300
Gordita Nacho Cheese - Chicken	270
Gordita Nacho Cheese - Steak	270
Chalupa	
Chalupa Supreme - Beef	390
Chalupa Supreme - Chicken	370
Chalupa Supreme - Steak	370
Chalupa Baja - Beef	430
Chalupa Baja - Chicken	400
Chalupa Baja - Steak	400
Chalupa Nacho Cheese - Beef	380
Chalupa Nacho Cheese - Chicken	350
Chalupa Nacho Cheese - Steak	350
Burritos	
Bean	370

TACO BELL

7-Layer	530
Chili Cheese	390
Burrito Supreme® - Beef	440
Burrito Supreme® - Chicken	410
Burrito Supreme® - Steak	420
Fiesta Burrito - Beef	390
Fiesta Burrito - Chicken	370
Fiesta Burrito - Steak	370
Grilled Stuft Burrito - Beef	730
Grilled Stuft Burrito - Chicken	680
Grilled Stuft Burrito - Steak	680

Specialties

Tostada	250
Mexican Pizza	550
Enchirito® - Beef	380
Enchirito® - Chicken	350
Enchirito® - Steak	360
MexiMelt®	290
Taco Salad w/Salsa	790
Taco Salad w/Salsa without shell	420
Express Taco Salad w/chips	620
Cheese Quesadilla	490
Chicken Quesadilla	540
Steak Quesadilla	540
Zesty Chicken Border Bowl™	730
Zesty Chicken Border Bowl™ without dressing	500
Southwest Steak Bowl	700

Nachos & Sides

Nachos	320
Nachos Supreme	450
Nachos BellGrande®	780
Pintos 'n Cheese	180
Mexican Rice	210
Cinnamon Twists	160

Breakfast

Breakfast Gordita	380
Breakfast Burrito	510
Breakfast Steak Burrito	500
Breakfast Quesadilla	400
Breakfast Steak Quesadilla w/Green Sauce	460

Sauces & Condiments

Border Sauce - Mild	5
Border Sauce - Hot	10
Border Sauce - Fire	15
Red Sauce	10
Green Sauce	10
Nacho Cheese Sauce	50
Pepper Jack Cheese Sauce	70
Fiesta Salsa	5
Sour Cream	45

TACO BELL – TACO JOHN'S

Guacamole	35
Cheddar Cheese	30
Three Cheese Blend	250
Creamy Lime Sauce	90
Creamy Jalapeno Sauce	70
Zesty Dressing	240

Taco John's

Tacos	Calories
Chicken Softshell Taco	200
Crispy Taco	190
Sierra Taco™ - Beef	500
Sierra Taco™ - Chicken	470
Softshell Taco	230
Taco Bravo®	360
Taco Burger	280

Burritos

Bean Burrito	380
Beefy Burrito	440
Chicken & Potato Burrito	470
Combination Burrito	410
Meat & Potato Burrito	500
Super Burrito	450

Specialties

Cheese Quesadilla	480
Chicken Festiva Salad	680
Chicken Festiva Salad w/o Dressing	390
Chicken Quesadilla	530
Chicken Super Nachos	860
Chicken Taco Salad	910
Chicken Taco Salad w/o Dressing	620
Potato Olés® Bravo	570
Super Nachos	900
Super Potato Olés®	970
Taco Salad	770
Taco Salad w/o dressing	600

Platters

Beef & Bean Chimi Platter	740
Beef Enchilada Platter	800
Chicken Enchilada Platter	710
Smothered Burrito Platter	850

Sides

Mexican Rice	250
Nachos	440
Potato Olés® - Kid's Meal	310
Potato Olés® - Large 9	790
Potato Olés® - Medium	620
Potato Olés® - Small	440
Refried Beans	360
Side Salad	290

TACO JOHN'S – TACO TIME

Texas Style Chili	280
Desserts	
Apple Grande	260
Choco Taco	310
Churros	160
Taco John's Cinnamon Mint Swirl (1)	10
Taco John's Cookies (Kid's Meal - 1 bag)	130
Limited Time Promotions	
Crunchy Chicken Burrito	630
Crunchy Chicken Caesar Salad	520
Crunchy Chicken Festiva Salad w/dressing	650
Crunchy Chicken Salad Festiva w/o dressing	470
Crunchy Chicken Side	460
Crunchy Chicken Taco Salad w/o dressing	600
Crunchy Chicken Taco Salad w/dressing	700
Local Favorites	
Bean Tostada	160
Cheese Crisp	220
Chicken Fajita Burrito	350
Chicken Festiva Burrito	570
Chilito	440
Double Enchilada	750
El Grande Burrito	730
El Grande Chicken Burrito	680
El Grande Chicken Taco	360
El Grande Taco	480
Mexi Rolls®	460
Potato Olés® w/nacho cheese	530
Ranch Burrito - Beef	440
Ranch Burrito - Chicken	410
Sierra Chicken Sandwich	480
Smothered Burrito	520
Taco John's Mexican Pizza	560
Tostada	200

Taco Time

Burritos	Calories
Beef, Bean, & Cheese	620
Big Juan Beef	640
Big Juan Chicken	620
Casita	650
Chicken & Black Bean	400
Chicken BLT	580
Crisp Bean	430
Crisp Chicken	420
Crisp Meat	550
Soft Bean	380
Soft Meat	490
Veggie	490

TACO TIME – TIM HORTON

Tacos
1/2 lb. Chicken Soft Taco	385
1/2 lb. Soft taco	510
Crisp Taco	295
Soft Taco	315
Super Soft Taco	510

Salads
Chicken Fiesta	390
Chicken Taco	370
Taco (Regular)	480
Tostada	630
Nachos	
Cheddar Melt	205
Nachos	680
Nachos Deluxe	1050
Taco Cheeseburger	635

Sides
Cheddar Fries (Large)	705
Cheddar Fries (Medium)	505
Cheddar Fries (Small)	350
Mexi-Fries (Large)	530
Mexi-Fries (Medium)	390
Mexi-Fries (Small)	265
Mexi-Rice	160
Refritos (cheese, sauce, chips)	325
Stuffed Fries (Large)	990
Stuffed Fries (Medium)	640
Stuffed Fries (Small)	490

Dessert
Cinnamon Crustos	375
Fruit-Filled Empanada	250

Sauces
Thousand Island Dressing	120
Green	5
Original Hot	10
Salsa Fresca	65

Tim Horton

DoNuts
	Calories
Angel Cream	280
Apple Fritter	300
Blueberry	220
Boston Cream	230
Canadian Maple	230
Chocolate Chip	230
Chocolate Glazed	350
Dutchie	280
Glazed	270
Honey Dip	230
Honey Stick	280

TIM HORTON

Maple Dip	250
Plain	220
Sour Cream Plain	280
Strawberry	220
Sugar Twist	230
Walnut Crunch	320

Timbits

Banana Cream	45
Chocolate Glazed	70
Dutchie	60
Honey Dip	50
Lemon	50
Plain	45
Spiced Apple	50
Strawberry	50

Muffins

Blueberry Bran	300
Carrot Whole Wheat	410
Chocolate Chip	390
Low-Fat Carrot	260
Low-Fat Cranberry	260
Low-Fat Honey	290
Oatbran Carrot 'n' Raisin	340
Oatbran 'n' Apple	350
Oatmeal Raisin	430
Raisin Bran	360
Wild Blueberry	330

Bagels

Blueberry	300
Cinnamon Raisin	300
Everything	300
Multigrain	300
Onion	295
Plain	290
Poppy Seed	300
Sesame Seed	300
Whole Wheat & Honey	300

Baked Goods

Cheese Croissant	240
Cherry Cheese Danish	380
Cranberry Biscuit	470
Croissant	210
Raisin Tea Biscuit	250
Raspberry Biscuit	470
Tea Biscuit	220

Cream Cheese

Garden Vegetable	150
Light	90
Plain	140
Strawberry	150

Cookies
Chocolate Chip	150
Oatcakes	190
Oatmeal Raisin	150
Peanut Butter	170
Peanut Butter Chocolate Chunk	170
Plain Macaroon	140

Beverages
Café Mocha	250
Cappuccino Ice	430
English Toffee Cappuccino	130
French Vanilla Cappuccino	130
Hot Chocolate	200

Sandwiches
Albacore Tuna Salad	350
Black Forest Ham & Swiss	640
Chunky Chicken Salad	380
Fireside Roast Beef	470
Garden Vegetable	460
Harvest Turkey Breast	470

Soup (10 oz)
Chicken Noodle	100
Chili	320
Cream of Broccoli	190
Cream of Mushroom	1950
Hearty Vegetable	130
Minestrone	125
Potato Bacon	195
Turkey & Wild Rice	120
Vegetable Beef Barley	110

Pies, Cakes, & Tarts
Apple Pie (1/4 pie)	540
Banana Cream Pie (1/4 pie)	440
Black Forest Cake (1/8 cake)	500
Celebration Cake (1/8 cake)	500
Cherry Pie (1/4 pie)	570
Chocolate Cream Pie (1/4 pie)	490
Chocolate Fantasy Cake (1/8 cake)	420
Raisin Butter Tart	330
Shadow Cake (1/8 cake)	430
Strawberry Tart	220

Togo's

Sandwiches (Regular)
	Calories
Albacore Tuna	450
Avocado & Cucumber	590
Avocado & Turkey	670
BBQ Beef	530
Black Forest Ham & Cheese	630
California Roasted Chicken	620

TOGO'S

Cheese	660
Chunky Chicken & Almond Salad	750
Egg Salad & Cheese	650
French Onion Dip	640
Hot or Cold Roast Beef	680
Hot Pastrami	810
Hummus	790
Meatballs In Zesty Tomato Sauce	690
Pastrami Reuben	650
Salami & Cheese	760
Savory BBQ Chicken	520
Sicilian Chicken	670
The Italian	740
Turkey & Bacon Club	600
Turkey & Cheese	600
Turkey, Ham & Cheese	600
Turkey, Roast Beef, & Cheese	670

Sandwiches (Large)

Albacore Tuna	800
Avocado & Cucumber	880
Avocado & Turkey	1000
BBQ Beef	780
Black Forest Ham & Cheese	920
California Roasted Chicken	1030
Cheese	930
Chunky Chicken & Almond Salad	1130
Egg Salad & Cheese	950
French Onion Dip	680
Hot or Cold Roast Beef	1030
Hot Pastrami	1170
Hummus	1170
Meatballs In Zesty Tomato Sauce	1060
Pastrami Reuben	970
Salami & Cheese	1110
Savory BBQ Chicken	780
Sicilian Chicken	1030
The Italian	1060
Turkey & Bacon Club	900
Turkey & Cheese	860
Turkey, Ham & Cheese	860
Turkey, Roast Beef, & Cheese	950

Salads

Farmer's Market	110
Oriental Chicken	370
Roasted Chicken Caesar	320
Taco	1020

Soup (Regular)

Baked Potato	290
Black Bean	180
Broccoli Cheese	180

Chicken Noodle	160
Chicken w/Wild Rice	340
Chili	140
New England Clam Chowder	140
Turkey Pot Pie Soup	180
Soup (Large)	
Baked Potato	440
Black Bean	270
Broccoli Cheese	270
Chicken Noodle	240
Chicken w/Wild Rice	510
Chili	200
New England Clam Chowder	200
Turkey Pot Pie Soup	270
Dressing (1 pouch) & Sides	
Caesar Dressing	240
Low Fat Balsamic Vinegrette Dressing	100
Oriental Sesame Dressing	240
Potato Salad (Regular)	230
Potato Salad (single)	170
Ranch Dressing	200
Sesame Orange Ginger Dressing	330

Wendy's

Sandwiches	**Calories**
Classic Single® w/ Everything	410
Big Bacon Classic®	570
Jr. Hamburger	270
Jr. Cheeseburger	310
Jr. Bacon Cheeseburger	380
Jr. Cheeseburger Deluxe	350
Hamburger - Kids' Meal	270
Cheeseburger - Kids' Meal	310
Grilled Chicken Sandwich	300
Chicken Breast Fillet Sandwich	430
Chicken Club Sandwich	470
Spicy Chicken Sandwich	430
Sandwich Components	
Hamburger Patty – 1/4 lb.	200
Hamburger Patty – 2 oz.	100
Grilled Chicken Fillet	110
Breaded Chicken Fillet	230
Spicy Chicken Fillet	230
Kaiser Bun	200
Sandwich Bun	160
American Cheese	70
American Cheese, Jr.	45
Bacon	20
Honey Mustard Sauce	25

WENDY'S

Salads

Caesar Side Salad	70
Homestyle Garlic Croutons - 1 pack	70
Side Salad	35
Chicken BLT Salad	310
Homestyle Garlic Croutons - 1 pack	70
Mandarin Chicken™ Salad	150
Roasted Almonds - 1 pack	130
Crispy Rice Noodles - 1 pack	60
Spring Mix Salad	180
Honey Roasted Pecans - 1 pack	130
Taco Supremo Salad	360
Taco Chips - 1 pack	220
Sour Cream - 1 pack	60
Salsa (1 each)	30

Dressings (1 pack)

Blue Cheese	260
Caesar Dressing	150
Creamy Ranch	230
Fat-Free French Style	80
House Vinaigrette Dressing	190
Honey Mustard Dressing	280
Low-Fat Honey Mustard	110
Oriental Sesame Dressing	250
Reduced Fat Creamy Ranch	100

French Fries

Kids' Meal	250
Medium	390
Biggie®	440
Great Biggie®	530

Stuffed Baked Potatoes

Plain	310
Bacon & Cheese	580
Broccoli & Cheese	480
Sour Cream & Chives	370
Whipped Margarine (1 pack)	60

Chili

Small	200
Large	300
Cheddar Cheese, 2 Tblsp shredded	70
Saltine Crackers (2)	25
Hot Chili Seasoning 1 pack	5

Crispy Chicken Nuggets

5 Piece	220
4 Piece Kids' Meal	180
Barbecue Sauce 1 pack	40
Honey Mustard Sauce 1 pack	130
Sweet & Sour Sauce 1 pack	45

Frosty

Junior	170

	Calories
Small	330
Medium	440

Whataburger

Sandwiches	Calories
Grilled Chicken	475
Honey Dijon Whatachick'n	720
Justaburger	310
Kids Justaburger	305
Triple Meat Whataburger	1110
Whataburger Jr	315
Whataburger Jr	610
Whataburger w/Bacon & Cheese	810
Whatacatch	470
Whatacatch, 2 pieces	815
Whatachick'n	525
Double Meat Whataburger	860
Other Items	
Chicken Strips, 2 pieces	380
Chicken Strips, 3 pieces	575
Chicken Strips, 4 pieces	765
Grilled Chicken Fajita Taco	365
Kids Chicken Strips	380
Salads	
Chicken Strips	420
Chicken Strips w/cheddar cheese	600
Chicken Strips w/cheese & bacon	675
Garden	50
Garden w/Cheddar cheese	215
Garden w/cheese & bacon	290
Grilled Chicken	230
Grilled Chicken w/Cheddar cheese	400
Grilled Chicken w/cheese & bacon	470
Seasoned Croutons (1 pack)	35
Dressings (1 Pack)	
Low Fat Ranch	65
Low Fat Vinaigrette	35
Ranch	310
Thousand Island	150
Salad Dressing (large sandwich)	55
Salad Dressing (small sandwich)	30
Sides	
American Cheese Slice (large sandwich)	90
American Cheese Slice (small sandwich)	45
Bacon (breakfast & small Sandwich)	75
Bacon (large sandwich)	110
Fries, large	515
Fries, medium	385
Fries, small	260
Gravy for Chicken Strips	50

WHATABURGER

Onion Rings, large	305
Onion Rings, medium	200
Breakfast	
Biscuit w/bacon	375
Biscuit w/bacon, egg & cheese	520
Biscuit w/egg & cheese	445
Biscuit w/sausage	515
Biscuit w/sausage gravy	490
Biscuit w/sausage, egg & cheese	660
Biscuit	300
Breakfast Platter w/bacon	700
Breakfast Platter w/sausage	840
Breakfast On A Bun w/bacon	400
Breakfast On A Bun w/sausage	540
Breakfast On A Bun Ranchero w/bacon	405
Breakfast On A Bun Ranchero w/sausage	545
Cinnamon Roll	860
Egg Sandwich	320
Grape Jelly	35
Hashbrown Sticks	140
Honey (1 pack)	25
Margarine (1 pack)	25
Pancake Syrup (1 pack)	120
Pancakes	615
Pancakes w/bacon	690
Pancakes w/sausage	830
Strawberry Jam (1 pack)	40
Taquito w/bacon & egg	390
Taquito w/bacon, egg & cheese	430
Taquito w/potato & egg	380
Taquito w/potato, egg & cheese	430
Taquito w/sausage & egg	390
Taquito w/sausage, egg & cheese	435
Texas Toast	330
Beverages	
Chocolate Shake, Kids	450
Chocolate Shake, Large	1215
Chocolate Shake, Medium	905
Chocolate Shake, Small	615
Strawberry Shake, Kids	450
Strawberry Shake, Large	1160
Strawberry Shake, Medium	910
Strawberry Shake, Small	620
Vanilla Shake, Kids	410
Vanilla Shake, Large	1120
Vanilla Shake, Medium	835
Vanilla Shake, Small	560
Orange Juice	140
Desserts	
Cookie, Chocolate Chunk	210

Cookie, Oatmeal Raisin	185
Cookie, Peanut Butter	215
Cookie, White Chocolate Macadamia Nut	230
Hot Apple Pie	240

White Castle

Item	Calories
Hamburger	140
Cheeseburger	160
Double Hamburger	240
Double Cheeseburger	290
Bacon Cheeseburger	200
Fish Sandwich	180
Chicken Sandwich	200
Breakfast Sandwich	340
Chicken Rings	215
Onion Rings	600
French Fries, Small	115
Cheese Sticks, 5	420
Shake, Vanilla	350
Shake, Chocolate	330

Winchells

Item	Calories
Glazed Rounds	230
Chocolate Rounds	240
Glazed Twist	230
Chocolate Twist	240
Chocolate Bar	240
Traditional Cake	215
Chocolate Iced Cake	230
Croissant	260

A&W

Sandwiches	Calories
Grilled Chicken	280
Hot Dogs	
Plain	280

Applebee's

Item	Calories
Bikini Banana Low Fat Strawberry Shortcake	230

Arby's

Roast Beef Sandwiches	Calories
Arby's Melt w/Cheddar	340
Junior Roast Beef	310
Regular Roast Beef	350
Market Fresh Salads (No Dressing)	
Caesar Salad	90
Caesar Side Salad	45
Grilled Chicken Caesar	230
Turkey Club Salad	350
Light Menu	
Light Grilled Chicken	280
Light Roast Chicken Deluxe	260
Light Roast Turkey Deluxe	260
Salads	
Garden	70
Grilled Chicken	210
Roast Chicken	160
Side	25
Side Items & Snacks	
Homestyle Fries Child-size	220
Potato Cakes (2)	250
Breakfast Items	
Biscuit With Bacon	320
Biscuit With Ham	330
Croissant With Bacon	300
Croissant With Ham	310
Sourdough With Ham	220
Sourdough With Sausage	330
Condiments	
Arby's Sauce® Packet	15
Au Jus Sauce	5
BBQ Dipping Sauce	40
BBQ Vinaigrette Dressing	140
Bronco Berry Sauce™	90
Buttermilk Ranch Dressing Reduced Cal.	60
Croutons – Cheese & Garlic	100
Croutons – Seasoned	30

151

LOWER CALORIES

ARBY'S – AU BON PAIN

French Toast Syrup	130
German Mustard Packet	5
Honey Mustard Sauce	130
Horsey Sauce® Packet	60
Italian Dressing — Reduced Calorie	25
Ketchup Packet	10
Marinara Sauce	35
Mayonnaise Packet	90
Mayonnaise Packet — Light, Cholesterol-Free	20

Au Bon Pain

Crossiants	Calories
Apple	220
Plain	250
Spinach & Cheese	250
Special Delights	
Oatmeal Bar	150
Bread & Rolls	
Baguette	120
Country White Sandwich Loaf	110
Multigrain Loaf	130
Parisienne	120
Petit Pain	200
Rosemary Garlic Bread Stick	200
Tomato Herb Loaf	140
Cream Cheese Spreads (2 oz. Serving)	
Veggie Or Walnut	140
Plain	120
Sun Dried Tomato	70
Sandwiches	
Thai Chicken	490
Sandwich Fillings	
Brie Cheese	150
Cambozola Cheese	200
Cheddar Cheese	170
Chicken Breast	120
Chicken Tarragon	210
Ham	150
Hummus	100
Provolone Cheese	140
Roast Beef	150
Swiss Cheese	160
Tuna Salad Mix	170
Turkey Breast	120
Salads	
Caesar	240
Charbroiled Salmon Filet w/yellow peppers	210
Chef	290
Chicken Caesar	310
Garden	160

AU BON PAIN

Mediterranean Chicken	230
Mozzarella & Red Pepper	360
Nicoise	350
Side Garden	90
Thai Chicken	260
Tomato, Mozzarella w/basil pesto	280
Salad Dressings (2 Tblsp)	
Balsamic Vinaigrette	190
Blue Cheese	130
Caesar	160
Fat Free Raspberry	35
Lite Honey Mustard	100
Lite Olive Oil Vinaigrette	60
Lite Ranch	110
Mediterranean	80
Parmesan & Peppercorn	170
Thai Peanut	70
Soups & Stews (8 oz.)	
Autumn Pumpkin	140
Baked Stuffed Potato	240
Beef	210
Black Bean	170
Broccoli Cheddar	230
Chicken Chili	210
Chicken Florentine	170
Chicken Noodle	90
Chicken Stew	230
Clam Chowder	220
Classic Chili w/beans	190
Corn & Green Chili Bisque	160
Corn Chowder	240
Curried Rice And Lentil	100
French Moroccan Tomato Lentil	110
French Onion	80
Garden Vegtable	40
Lobster Bisque	250
Mediterrean Pepper	190
Mediterrean Seafood	170
Old Fashoned Tomato	130
Pasta E Fagiolo	160
Potato Cheese	180
Potato Leek	190
Red Beans, Rice & Sausage	180
Southern Black Eyed Pea	190
Southwest Tortilla Soup	140
Southwest Vegetable	150
Split Pea	140
Tomato Florentine	70
Turkey Chili	200
Tuscan Vegetable	130

LOWER CALORIES

Vegetable Beef Barley	80
Vegetarian Chili	170
Vegetarian Lentil	110
Vegetarian Minestrone	70
Wild Mushroom Bisque	110

Atlanta Bread Company

Bagels (4 oz.)	**Calories**
Everything	310
Onion	300
Poppy Seed	310
Pumpernickel	300
Sesame Seed	310
Breads (2 oz.)	
Asiago	150
Braided Challah	150
Chocolate Craisin Bread	200
Cinnamon Raisin	170
Cracked Wheat	160
Focaccia	170
French	140
Honey Wheat	150
Nine Grain	150
Olive	180
Onion	160
Pecan Raisin Loaf	200
Pesto	150
Powerloaf Multiloaf	150
Pumpernickel	150
Rosemary Focaccia	190
Rye	150
Sourdough	140
Sundried Tomato	150
Tuscana Parmesan	160
Rolls (2.6 oz.)	
French	180
Sourdough	190
Salads	
Ceasar Salad	220
Chicken House	115
Fruit	140
Greek	120
Greek Chicken	210
House	35
Tuna	240
Sandwiches	
Honey Maple Ham	420
Turkey Breast	420
Veggie	290

ATLANTA BREAD CO.

Soups (1 Cup)

Baked Potato	210
Black Bean & Rice	110
Black Bean w/ Ham	200
Chicken Chili	220
Chicken Gumbo	110
Chicken 'n Dumpling	240
Chicken Noodle	110
Chicken Tortilla	140
Chili w/ Beans	280
Clam Chowder	270
Country Bean	140
Cream of Broccoli	150
French Onion	60
Garden Veggie	80
Italian Style Wedding	120
Lentil & Roasted Garlic	200
Mushroom Barley & Sage	75
Pasta Fagioli	160
Seven Bean w/ Ham	240
Southwest Chicken	180
Szechuan Hot & Sour	80
Tomato Florentine	120
Tomato, Fennel & Dill	100
Vegetable Chili	180
Wisconsin Cheese	210

Specialty Sweets (1)

Choc Macadamia Biscotti	140
Eclairs	140
Vanilla Almond Biscotti	130

Cream Cheeses (2 oz.)

Chive	190
Honey Walnut Raisin	200
Olive	180
Raspberry	180
Veggie	190

Smoothies (16 oz.)

Heath Coffee	235
Kona Mocha Coffee	235
Pineapple Mango Banana	220
Spiced Chai Tea	130
Strawberry Banana	250
Strawberry Banana Blueberry	240
Vanilla Cafechillo	235

Croissants (1)

Butter	300

Dressings

Thousand Island, 2 oz	140
Asian Sesame Ginger, 1 oz	128
Bleu Cheese, 2 oz	140

ATLANTA BREAD CO. – BACKYARD BURGERS

Caesar, 2 Tblsp	150
Dill Sauce, .25 oz	30
Fat Free Ranch, 2 Tblsp	20
Fat Free Raspberry Vinaigrette, 2 Tblsp	25
Fat Free Toasted Sesame, 2 Tblsp	50
Greek, 2 Tblsp	100
House Italian, 2 oz	100
Vinaigrette, 2 Tblsp	100

Auntie Anne's

Pretzels	Calories
Garlic Pretzel	320
Jalapeño Pretzel	270
Sour Cream & Onion Pretzel	310
Dipping Sauces	
Light Cream Cheese	70
Strawberry Cream Cheese	110
Caramel Dip	135
Cheese Sauce	100
Chocolate Flavored Dip	130
Marinara Sauce	10
Sweet Mustard	60
Hot Salsa Cheese	100
Dutch Ice®	
Grape Dutch Ice 14 fl. oz.	180
Kiwi-Banana Dutch Ice 14 fl. oz.	190
Blue Raspberry Dutch Ice 14 fl. oz.	175
Strawberry Dutch Ice 14 fl. oz.	220
Wild Cherry Dutch Ice 14 fl. oz.	230

Backyard Burgers

Classic Burgers	Calories
Great Little Burger	280
Back Yard Specialties	
Back Yard BLT	270
Back Yard Hot Dog	310
Gardenburger	140
Dipping Sauces	
Barbeque	50
Gourmet	150
Gravy	70
Honey Mustard	170
Chicken Sandwiches	
Barbeque Chicken Sandwich	280
Blackened Chicken Sandwich	290
Hawaiian Chicken Sandwich	280
Lemon Butter Chicken Sandwich	260
Savory Chicken Sandwich	230
Baked Potatoes And Fries	
Traditional Fries	190

BACKYARD BURGERS – BEN & JERRY'S

Garden Fresh Salads
Blackened Chicken Salad	160
Charbroiled Chicken Salad	140
Garden Fresh Salad	25

Salad Dressings
Fat-Free Honey Dijon	60
Fat-Free Italian	20
Fat-Free Ranch	60
Honey Mustard	140
Italian	200

Baja Fresh

Tacos	**Calories**
Baja Fish	270
Baja Mahi Mahi	260
Original Baja Style, Chicken	190
Original Baja Style, Shrimp	190
Original Baja Style, Steak	220
Salads	
Mahi Mahi Ensalada	280
Shrimp Ensalada	180
Side Salad	70
Sides	
Cebollitas	40
Dressing, Fat Free Salsa Verde	15
Guacamole, medium	110
Guacamole, small	70
Salsa	50

Baskin Robbins

Sherbets, Ices, Sorbets (Reg. Scoop)	**Calories**
Daiquiri Ice	130
Peachy Keen Sorbet	110
Rainbow Sherbet	160
Low-fat Ice Cream (Reg Scoop)	
Espresso 'n Cream	180
No Sugar Ice Cream (Reg Scoop)	
Peach Crumb Pie	180
Thin Mint	160
Soft Serve Non-fat Yougurt (Small)	
Chocolate 5 oz.	190
Truly Free Yougurt (Small)	
Café Mocha	140

Ben & Jerry's

Frozen Yogurt	**Calories**
Cherry Garcia®	170
Chocolate Fudge Brownie	190

BEN & JERRY'S – BOSTON MARKET

Single Containers

Cherry Garcia	220
Chocolate Fudge Brownie	230
Cookie Dough	240
Vanilla For a Change	200

Bojangles

Sandwiches — Calories

	Calories
Grilled Filet without mayo	235
Grilled Filet w/mayo	335

Individual Fixin'

Cajun Pintos	110
Marinated Cole Slaw	136
Corn On The Cob	140
Dirty Rice	166
Green Beans	25
Macaroni & Cheese	198
Potatoes w/o gravy	80

Snacks

Buffalo Bites	180

Boston Market

Entrees — Calories

	Calories
Dark Meat Chicken, no skin	190
White Meat Chicken, no skin or wing	170
White Meat Chicken, w/skin or wing	280
Grilled Chicken Teriyaki	290
Honey Glazed Ham (lean)	210
Marinated Grilled Chicken	230
Skinless Chicken Rotisserie Turkey Breast	170

Sides (1 serving)

Butternut Squash	150
Chicken Gravy	15
Fruit Salad	70
Green Bean Casserole	80
Green Beans	70
Jumpin Juice Squares	150
New Potatoes	130
Old-fashioned Potato Salad	200
Rice Pilaf	140
Savory Stuffing	190
Steamed Vegetables	30
Whole Kernal Corn	180

Soup (3/4 Cup)

Chicken Noodle	100
Chicken Tortilla (no toppings)	80
Chicken Tortilla (w/toppings)	170
Turkey Tortilla (no toppings)	70
Turkey Tortilla (w/toppings)	160

LOWER CALORIES

BRUSTER'S – CAPTAIN D'S

Bruster's

No Sugar Added, Fat-Free Ice Cream (1/2 Cup)	Calories
Chocolate	100
Chocolate Caramel Swirl	120
Chocolate Fudge Ripple	120
Chocolate Raspberry Swirl	110
Cinnamon	100
Vanilla	100
Vanilla Caramel Swirl	110
Vanilla Fudge Ripple	110
Vanilla Raspberry Swirl	110

Burger King

Breakfast	Calories
Croissant w/egg & cheese	320
Hash Brown Rounds, small	230
Burgers & Sandwiches	
Cheeseburger	360
Chicken Tenders 4 pieces	170
Chicken Tenders 5 pieces	210
Chicken Tenders 6 pieces	250
Chicken Whopper Jr. – no mayo	270
Hamburger	310
Veggie Burger	330
Veggie Burger w/reduced-fat mayo	290
Whopper Jr.– no mayo	310
Whopper Jr. w/cheese – no mayo	360
Sides	
Chili	190
Onion Rings, small	180
Salads	
Chicken Caesar – no dressing or croutons	160
Side Garden – no dressing	25

Captain D's

Item	Calories
Broiled Chicken Breast	102
Broiled Fish Lunch	435
Broiled Shrimp Lunch	421
Gumbo	172
Stuffed Crab	91
Side Items	
Breadstick	113
Cheesesticks	218
Cocktail Sauce	137
Cocktail Sauce	34
Cole Slaw	158
Crackers	50

LOWER CALORIES

CAPTAIN D'S – CHICK-FIL-A

Cracklins	218
Dressings	
Blue Cheese	105
French	111
Honey Mustard	160
Light Italian	16
Ranch	92
Other	
Green Beans (seasoned)	46
Imitation Sour Cream	29
Margarine	102
Rice	124
Salad	20
Slice of Cheese	54
Sweet & Sour Sauce	52
Tartar Sauce	75
Vegetable Medley	36
White Beans	126

Caribou

Item	Calories
2% Capp, 12 oz	122
2% Capp, 16 oz	162
2% Capp, 20 oz	203
2% Chai Latte, 12 oz	215
2% Latte, 12 oz	129
2% Latte, 16 oz	171
2% Latte, 20 oz	214
Chocolate Cooler, 12 oz	193
Coffee Cooler, 12 oz	173
Espresso Cooler, 12 oz	136
Espresso Cooler, 16 oz	193
Skim Capp, 12 oz	84
Skim Capp, 16 oz	113
Skim Capp, 20 oz	141
Skim Chai, 12 oz	177
Skim Latte, 12 oz	91
Skim Latte, 16 oz	121
Skim Latte, 20 oz	152
Skim Mocha, 12 oz	226
Straw Ban Smoothie, 12 oz	190
Vanilla Cooler, 12 oz	193
Wild Berry Smoothie, 12 oz	176

Chick-Fil-A

Breakfast	Calories
Biscuit & Gravy	310
Biscuit w/bacon	300
Biscuit w/bacon & egg	390

CHICK-FIL-A – CHURCH'S

Biscuit w/egg	340
Biscuit w/egg & cheese	390
Hashbrowns	170

Sandwiches & Specialties

Chargrilled Chicken Deluxe Sandwich	280
Chargrilled Chicken Filet – no bun or pickle	100
Chargrilled Chicken Sandwich	280
Chargrilled Chicken Sandwich – no butter	240
Chicken Filet – no bun or pickle	230
Chicken Soup (1 cup)	100
Chick-N-Strips (4 count)	250
Nuggets (8 pack)	260

Salads

Chargrilled Chicken Garden	180
Chargrilled Chicken Caesar	240
Side Salad	80

Sides & Sauces (1 packet)

Carrot & Raisin Salad, Small	130
Croutons, Garlic & Butter	90
Barbeque Sauce	45
Dijon Honey Mustard Sauce	50
Honey Mustard Sauce	45
Polynesian Sauce	110
Sunflower Kernels, roasted	80

Dressing (1 packet)

Fat-Free Dijon Honey Mustard	60
Light Italian	20
Thousand Island	170

Drinks

Diet Lemonade, small	25
Iced Tea Sweet, small	80
Lemonade, small	170

Chuck E. Cheese

Pizza (2 Medium Slices)	Calories
Cheese	330

Salad Bar/Dressings (2 Tblsp)	
Catalina	35
Lite Ranch	80
Olive Oil & Vinegar	90
Thousand Island	110

Church's

Main Items	Calories
Breast – no batter or skin	145
Krispy Tender Strips (1 Strip)	137
Leg, fried	140
Leg – no batter or skin	118
Thigh, fried	230

Thigh – no batter or skin	180
Wing, fried	250
Wing – no batter or skin	160
Sides	
Cajun Rice, reg	130
Cole Slaw, reg	92
Collard Greens, reg	25
Corn on the Cob (1)	139
French Fries, reg	210
Macaroni & Cheese, reg	210
Mashed Potatoes & gravy, reg	90
Okra, Reg"	210
Whole Jalapeno Peppers (2)	10
Sauces (1 Package)	
BBQ	29
Creamy Jalapeno	102
Honey Mustard	111
Purple Pepper	46
Sweet & Sour	31

Dairy Queen

Cones	**Calories**
Chocolate Soft Serve, 1/2 Cup	150
Vanilla Soft Serve, 1/2 Cup	140
Malts, Shakes, Slushes	
Misty Slush, small	220
Novelties	
Chocolate Dilly Bar	210
DQ Sandwich	200
Fudge Bar – no sugar added	50
Lemon Freez'r	80
Starkiss	80
Vanilla Orange Bar – no sugar added	60
Sandwich & Sides	
BBQ Pork Sandwich	280
Cheeseburger	340
Chili'n'Cheese Dog	330
Grilled Chicken Salad w/Fat-Free Italian	230
Grilled Chicken Sandwich	310
Hamburger	290
Hot Dog	240

Del Taco

Tacos	**Calories**
Chicken Soft Taco	210
Soft Taco	160
Taco	160
Ultimate Taco	260

DEL TACO – DENNY'S

Burritos

Bean & Cheese Green Burrito	280
Bean & Cheese Red Burrito	270

Salads

Taco Salad	350

Burgers

Cheeseburger	330
Hamburger	280

Sides

Rice (cup)	140

Fries

Small Fries	210

Breakfast

Breakfast Burrito	250
Side of Bacon (2 slices)	50

Denny's

Breakfast	**Calories**
Bacon, 4 Strips"	162
Bagel, Dry"	235
Belgian Waffle	304
Egg Beaters, Egg Substitute"	71
Egg, One"	120
English Muffin, Dry"	125
Grits	80
Ham, Grilled Slice"	94
Hashed Browns, Plain"	218
Toast, dry)	90
Topping, blueberry	106
Topping, cherry	86
Topping, strawberry	115

Sides

Applesauce	60
Baked Potatoe, plain w/skin	220
Bread Stuffing, plain	100
Carrots In Honey Glaze	80
Corn in Butter Sauce	120
Cottage Cheese	72
Green Beans w/bacon	60
Green Peas w/butter sauce	100
Mashed Potatoes, plain"	105
Sliced Tomatoes (3)	13
Vegetable Rice Pilaf	85

Entrees

Fried Shrimp Dinner	219
Grilled Chicken Breast Dinner	130
Pot Roast Dinner w/gravy	292
Shrimp Scampi Skillet Dinner	289

Salads

Garden Deluxe w/Chicken Breast	264
Side Garden, no dressing	113

Soup

Chicken Noodle	60
Vegetable Beef	79

Einstein Brothers Bagel

Bagels	**Calories**
Lucky Green	320
Chopped Onion	330
Cinnamon Sugar	330
Dark Pumpernickel	320
Honey Whole Wheat	320
Jalapeno	330
Plain	320
Pumpkin	330
Salt	330
Sun-Dried Tomato	320

Bread Specialty

Bagel Mini Shtick Corn Meal	170
Bagel Mini ShtickSesame	180
Bagel Twist	220

Specialty Coffee

Americano, regular (basically zero)	0
Americao, large (basically zero)	0
Cafe Latte, regular	140
Caffe Latte – non-fat, large	180
Caffe Latte – non-fat, medium	140
Caffe Latte – non-fat, regular"	100
Cappuccino, medium	190
Cappuccino – non-fat, regular"	60
Cappuccino, large (w/low-fat milk)	150
Cappuccino, medium (w/low-fat milk)	130
Cappuccino, regular	90
Chai Skim Milk, regular	190
Espresso, regular	1
Low-Fat Mocha, regular	190

Iced Specialty Coffee

Iced Americano, 8 oz (basically zero)	0
Iced Coffee, regular	0
Iced Latte, medium	120
Iced Non-Fat Latte, medium	90
Low-Fat Iced Mocha, medium	180
Low-Fat Mocha, regular	190

Cold Beverages

Apple Juice Box	120
Fruit Punch Juice Box	90
Half & Half	40
Iced Tea, Unsweetened (basically zero)	0

EINSTEIN BROTHERS BAGEL

Low-Fat 2% Milk	120
Minute Maid Country Style OJ	100
Minute Maid Orange	106
Minute Maid Orig. Style Lemonade	96
Minute Maid Premium Orange Juice	110
Nestea Peach Iced Tea	78
Nestea Raspberry Iced Tea	78
Nestea Southern Style Iced Tea	123
Nestea Unsweetened Iced Tea (basically zero)	0
Odwalla Fresh Squeezed Orange Juice	143
Cream Cheese (2 Tblsp)	
Whipped Blueberry	70
Whipped Cappuccino	70
Whipped Garden Vegetable	60
Whipped Honey Almond Reduced-Fat	70
Whipped Jalapeno Salsa	60
Whipped Maple Raisin Walnut	60
Whipped Onion And Chive	70
Whipped Plain	70
Whipped Plain Reduced Fat	60
Whipped Pumpkin	100
Whipped Smoked Salmon	60
Whipped Strawberry	70
Whipped Sundried Tomato & Basil	60
Hot Tea	
Cinnamon Apple Spice	0
Earl Grey	0
English Breakfast	0
Lemon Zinger	0
Mandarin Orange Spice	0
Peppermint	0
Retail Food	
Fruit And Yogurt Parfait	190
Kettle Classic Natural Potato Chips	100
Tortilla Strips	140
Salad Dressings	
Asian Sesame	80
Caesar	150
Chipotle BBQ	110
Honey Chipotle Dressing	140
Horseradish Sauce Dressing	170
Raspberry Vinaigrette	160
Thousand Island	110
Wasabi Oriental Dressing	80
Salad Extras	
Bagel Croutons	25
Sweet Roasted Walnuts	180
Salads	
Chicken Salad Salad On Greens	210
Egg Salad	200

EINSTEIN BROTHERS BAGEL

Fresh Fruit Cup	110
Mixed Greens	220
Roasted Corn Salad	90
Tuna Salad	150
Tuna Salad Salad on Greens	170
Sandwich Fillings	
American Cheese (1 slice)	70
Cheddar Cheese (1 slice)	80
Pepper Jack Cheese (1 slice)	100
Peppered Bacon (3 slices)	90
Provolone Cheese (1 slice)	70
Smoked Salmon, Port Chatham (2 oz)	110
Smoked Salmon, Sea Specialties (2 oz)	92
Swiss Cheese (1 slice)	80
Sandwich, Assembled	
Egg, Original	480
Ham	450
Roast Beef	460
Smoked Turkey	420
The Veg Out	490
Tuna Salad	470
Turkey Pastrami Deli	440
Bread Sandwiches on 12-Grain	
Deli Chicken Salad	440
Deli Tuna Salad	440
Challah Deli Sandwiches	
Deli Egg Salad	430
Deli Tuna Salad	370
BBQ Chicken Sandwich	380
Roasted Chicken & Smoked Gouda	440
Soups	
Broccoli, Sharp Cheddar (cup)	230
Chicken & Wild Rice (cup)	190
Chicken Noodle (cup)	220
Clam Chowda (cup)	160
Low Fat Minestroni (cup)	180
Tomoato Bisque (cup)	190
Tortilla Soup (bowl)	200
Tortilla Soup (cup)	90
Turkey Chili (cup)	140
Spreads	
Butter (1 Tblsp)	100
Butter And Margarine Blend Spread (1 Tblsp)	60
Fruit Spread, Apricot (1 oz)	75
Fruit Spread, Grape (1 oz)	75
Fruit Spread, Grape (1 oz)	75
Fruit Spread, Strawberry (1 oz)	75
Honey Butter (1 Tblsp)	90
Hummus, Retail (12 oz)	110
Peanut Butter, Creamy (2 Tblsp)	190

EINSTEIN BROTHERS BAGEL – GODFATHER'S PIZZA

Choose Two: Half Salads
Asian Chicken	234
Caesar Side	220

Half Sandwiches On Bagel
Half Ham	227
Half Roast Beef	234
Half Smoked Turkey	213
Half Turkey Pastrami	225

Half Sandwiches On 12-Grain
Half Chicken Salad	244
Half Tuna Salad	213

Half Challah Sandwiches
Half Chicken Salad	211
Half EBBQ Chicken Sandwich	196
Half Egg Salad	218
Half Roasted Chicken & Smoked Gouda	231

Fazoli's

Italian Specialties	Calories
Baked Ziti	490
Cheese Ravioli w/Marinara	480
Pastas	
Spaghetti w/Marinara	420
Spaghetti w/Meat Sauce	450
Breadsticks	
1 Breadstick	140
1 Breadstick – dry	90
Soups And Salads	
Chicken Finger Salad	190
Garden Salad	30
Honey French Dressing	150
House Italian Dressing	110
Minestrone Soup	120
Ranch Dressing	150
Reduced Calorie Italian Dressing	50
Thousand Island Dressing	130

Godfather's Pizza

Medium-Original (1 slice)	Calories
Cheese	260
Hawaiian	280
Pepperoni	290
Veggie	280
Large-Original (1 slice)	
Cheese	290
Hawaiian	320
Pepperoni	330
Veggie	310

GODFATHER'S PIZZA – HARDEE'S

Medium-Golden Crust (1 slice)

All Meat Combo	300
Bacon Cheeseburger	240
Cheese	220
Combo	290
Hawaiian	240
Pepperoni	260
Taco	290
Veggie	230

Large-Golden Crust (1 slice)

All Meat Combo	350
Bacon Cheeseburger	330
Cheese	250
Combo	330
Hawaiian	270
Pepperoni	290
Taco	340
Veggie	260

Medium-Thin Crust (1 slice)

All Meat Combo	280
Bacon Cheeseburger	250
Cheese	200
Combo	270
Hawaiian	220
Pepperoni	230
Taco	270
Veggie	210

Large-Thin Crust (1 slice)

All Meat Combo	310
Bacon Cheeseburger	290
Cheese	220
Combo	290
Hawaiian	230
Pepperoni	250
Taco	300
Veggie	230

Hardee's

Chicken	Calories
Chicken Strips (3)	120
Chicken Strips (5)	200
Fried Chicken Leg	170
Fried Chicken Wing	200
Sides	
Cole Slaw (Small)	240
Gravy	20
Mashed Potatoes (Small)	70
Burgers & Sandwiches	
BBQ Grilled Chicken Sandwich	270
Cheeseburger	315

HARDEE'S – KRYSTAL

Hamburger	265
Hot Ham 'N' Cheese™ Sandwich	305
Regular Roast Beef Sandwich	310
Slammer	270
Slammer w/cheese	320
Breakfast	
Apple Cinnamon 'N' Raisin™ Biscuit	250
Cinammon 'N' Raisin™ Biscuit	250
Made from Scratch® Biscuit (no margarine)	360
Made from Scratch® Biscuit (w/margarine)	390
Regular Hash Rounds™ Potatoes (16)	230

Jamba Juice

Juices (16 oz.)	Calories
Carrot	100
Orange	220
Orange/Banana	220
Orange/Carrot	160
Vibrant-C	210
Wheatgrass (1 oz.)	5
Baked Goods	
Grin'n'Carrot	250
Pizza Protein Stick	230

KFC

Chicken	Calories
Extra Crispy – Drumstick	160
Extra Crispy – Whole Wing	190
Hot & Spicy – Drumstick	140
Hot & Spicy – Whole Wing	180
Original – Drumstick	140
Original – Whole Wing	145
Sandwiches	
Honey BBQ Flavor	310
Original Recipe – no sauce	360
Tender Roast – no sauce	270
Tender Roast w/sauce	350
Sides	
Corn on the Cob	150
Green Beans	45
Mashed Potatoes w/gravy	120
Mean Greens	70

Krystal

Item	Calories
Apple Turnover	220
Chili	200
Corn Pup	260
Hash Browns	190

Krystal	160
Krystal Chik	240
Krystal, Bacon & Cheese	190
Krystal, Cheese	180
Krystal, Double	260
Pup, Chili Cheese	210
Pup, Plain	170
Sunriser	240

Little Ceasar's

Pizza by The Slice	Calories
12" Round Pizza (1 slice)	
Cheese Only	167
Pepperoni	190
14" Round Pizza (1 slice)	
Cheese Only	180
Veggie	199
12" Thin Crust (1 slice)	
Cheese Only	141
Pepperoni	150
14" Thin Crust (1 slice)	
Cheese Only	140
Pepperoni	164
16" Round Pizza (1 slice)	
Cheese Only	193
Sides	
Crazy Bread (1 stick)	98
Crazy Sauce	45
Salads	
Tossed Side	50
Antipasto	175
Dressings	
Fat-Free Italian	15

Long John Silvers

Sides & Starters	Calories
Cheesesticks (3)	140
Corn Cobbette (1)	90
Crumblies	170
Rice	180

McDonald's

Sandwiches	Calories
Cheeseburger	330
Hamburger	280
Chicken McNuggets/Sauces	
Chicken McNuggets® (4-piece)	210
Barbeque Sauce	45

MCDONALD'S – PANERA BREAD

Honey	45
Honey Mustard Sauce	50
Hot Mustard Sauce	60
Light Mayonnaise	45
Sweet 'N Sour Sauce	50
Salads	
Bacon Ranch (without chicken)	140
Butter Garlic Croutons	50
Caesar (without chicken)	90
California Cobb (without chicken)	160
Side	15
Salad Dressings	
Newman's Own® Cobb	120
Newman's Own® Light Balsamic Vinaigrette	90
Breakfast	
Bagel (plain)	260
English Muffin	150
Hash Browns	130
Sausage Breakfast Burrito	290
Scrambled Eggs (2)	160

Miami Subs

Salads	Calories
Greek	285
Greek Side w/dressing	79

Nathan's Famous

Item	Calories
Hot Dog	310
Hot Dog Nuggets (6)	350

Old Spaghetti Factory

Item	Calories
Spaghetti w/mushroom sauce	450
Spaghetti w/mushroom/meat sauce	490
Spaghetti w/mushroom/tomato sauce	450
Spaghetti w/tomato sauce	440
Spaghetti w/tomato/meat sauce	480
Salad Dressing	
Thousand Island, 1.5 oz	180
Balsamic Vinaigrette, 1 oz	160
Honey Mustard, 2 Tblsp	40

Panera Bread

Bagels	Calories
Nine Grain	290
Plain	290
Pumpkin	280

Breads (2 oz, unless noted)

Sourdough Roll (2.5 oz)	170
Sourdough Baguette, round or loaf	130
French Roll (2.25 oz)	160
French Loaf, extra-large loaf	130
French Baquette	140
Asiago Cheese Demi Loaf	150
Braided Challah	160
Three-Seed Demi	140
Olive Demi	140
Asiagio Cheese Focaccia	150
Rosemary & Onion Focaccia	140
Basil Pesto Focaccia	150
Rye Loaf	140
Nine-Grain	150
Honey Wheat	140
Sunflower Loaf	160
Tomato Basil, extra-large loaf	130
Cinnamon Raisin Loaf	160
Holiday Bread	150
Country Demi, Loaf, Miche	120
French Baguette, Miche	120
Multigrain Loaf, Miche	130
Sesame Semolina Demi, Loaf, Miche	130
Three Cheese Demi, Loaf, Miche	130
Stone Milled Rye Loaf, Miche	190
Kalamata Olive Demi, Loaf	140
Raisin Pecan boule	140

Sandwiches

Turkey on Sourdough	450
PB&J on French	440

Soups (8 oz)

Black Bean	180
Chicken Noodle	110
Garden Vegetable	100
Chicken Chili	180
Ginger Tomato Florentine	80
Moroccan Tomato Lentil	110
Potato Cream Cheese	190
Lentin	120
Gumbo	110
Tomato Bisque	160
Forest Mushroom	140
Santa Fe Roasted Corn	140
Corn & Green Chile Chowder	190
Creamy Country Asparagus	180
Farmers' Market Bisque	140
Fire Roasted Vegetable Bisque	180
Mesa Bean & Vegetable	100

Savory Vegetable Bean	120
Vegetable & Sirloin	100
Tomato Mushroom & Barley	110
Salads	
Strawberry Poppyseed	240
Spreads (2 oz)	
Plain Cream Cheese	190
Avg All Reduced-Fat Cream Cheese	135
Roasted Garlic Hummus	90
Muffins	
Banana Nut Muffie	290
Chocolate Chip Muffie	270
Pumpkin Muffie	270
Danish	
Coffee Cake-Cherry Cheese	190
Croissants	
Apple	340
Butter	310
Raspberry Cheese	320

Papa John's Pizza

Original Crust Pizza (1 slice of 14" Pizza)	**Calories**
Cheese	285
Chicken Alfredo	300
Garden Special	280
Pepperoni	305
Sausage	320
Spinach Alfredo	335
The Works	340
Thin Crust Pizza (1 slice of 14" Pizza)	
Cheese	235
Chicken Alfredo	270
Garden Special	225
Meat	395
Pepperoni	265
Sausage	285
Spinach Alfredo	295
The Works	320
Side Items	
BBQ	50
Bread Sticks	140
Buffalo	25
Cheese Sauce	60
Cheese Sticks	180
Chickenstrips	85
Cinnapie	115
Pizza Sauce	25
Ranch	140

Philly Connection

Sandwiches (Regular Size)	Calories
Steak	350
Lite, Grilled Chicken	290
Lite, Chicken Hoagie	290
Lite, Turkey Hoagie	280
Lite, Veggie Hoagie	260
Lite, Chicken Parmesan	330
Lite, Chicken Works	330
Salads	
Veggie Delite	220
Cheesesteak	320
Chicken Tenders	340
Grilled Chicken	140
Turkey	130
Tuna	290
Garden	40
Lite, Grilled Chicken	140
Lite, Turkey	130

Pizza Hut

Hand Tossed Pizza (1 slice)	Calories
Cheese	240
Beef	330
Ham	260
Pepperoni	280
Italian Sausage	340
Pork Topping	320
Meat Lover's	320
Veggie Lover's	220
Pepperoni Lover's	250
Supreme	270
Super Supreme	290
Chicken Supreme	230
Thin'n'Crispy Pizza (1 Slice)	
Cheese	200
Beef	270
Ham	170
Pepperoni	190
Italian Sausage	290
Pork Topping	270
Veggie Lover's	190
Pepperoni Lover's	250
Supreme	250
Super Supreme	280
Chicken Supreme	200
Pan Pizza (1 Slice)	
Cheese	290

Beef	330
Ham	260
Pepperoni	280
Italian Sausage	340
Pork Topping	320
Meat Lover's	360
Veggie Lover's	270
Pepperoni Lover's	330
Supreme	320
Super Supreme	340
Chicken Supreme	270
Stuffed Crust Pizza (1 Slice)	
Cheese	360
Beef	390
Ham	330
Pepperoni	360
Pork Topping	380
Veggie Lover's	340
Chicken Supreme	350
Chicago Dish Pizza (1 Slice)	
Pepperoni	390
Veggie Lover's	370
Big New Yorker Pizza (1 Slice)	
Pepperoni	390
Ham	370
Appetizers	
Mild Buffalo Wings (5)	200
Hot Buffalo Wings (4)	210
Garlic Bread (1 slice)	150
Breadstick (1)	130
Breadstick Dipping Sauce	30

Qdoba

Shells	Calories
Hard Taco	70
Soft Taco	95
Sides	
Tortilla Soup	80
Rice	200
Beans, Black or Pinto	130
Sour Cream	95
Non-fat Sour Cream	55
Fajita Vegetables	45
Meats	
Chicken	190
Steak	205
Ground Sirloin	205
Shredded Beef	215
Grilled Vegetables	50

Sauces

Ranchero	15
Poblano Pesto	65
Mole	60
Corn Bean	60
Picante Ranch Dressing	175

Quizno's

Sandwiches	Calories
Small Smoked Turkey w/Raspberry Chipolte Sauce	350
Small Honey Borboun Chicken	360
Small Turkey Lite	335

Sbarro

Item (1 Slice Or Serving)	Calories
Garlic Roll	180
Mixed Vegetables	170
Salad, Green Garden	50

Schlotzsky's

Sandwiches	Calories
Smoked Turkey Breast (small)	335
The Vegetarian (small)	325
Albacore Tuna (small)	335
Hot Sandwiches (where available)	
Dijon Chicken (small)	330
Santa Fe Chicken (small)	405
Pesto Chicken (small)	345
Corned Beef (small)	395
Roast Beef (small)	420
Western Vegetarian (small)	425
Vegetable Club (small)	370
BLT (small)	380
BLT (regular)	580
Turkey Guacamole (small)	425
Wraps	
Zesty Albacore Tuna	310
Deli Salads	
Fresh Fruit Salad	125
Fresh Fruit Salad (small)	85
Chicken & Pesto Pasta Salad (small)	325
Chicken Salad	375
Chicken Salad (small)	285
Albacore Tuna Salad	220
Albacore Tuna Salad (small)	135
Potato Salad	290
Mustard Potato Salad	250
Homestyle Cole Slaw	190

SCHLOTZSKY'S – SHONEY'S

Elbow Macaroni Salad	275
California Pasta Salad	60
Chicken Caesar	110
Caesar	30
Smoked Turkey Chef's	200
Garden	50
Small Garden	25
Chinese Chicken	130
Greek	160
Ham & Turkey Chef's	200
Salad Extras	
Light Spicy Ranch	140
Light Italian	90
Greek Balsamic Vinaigrette	170
Sesame Ginger Vinaigrette	170
Chow Mein Noodles	75
Garlic Cheese Croutons	45
Bread	
Sourdough Bun (small)	225
Wheat Bun (small)	225
Dark Rye Bun (small)	220
Jalapeño Cheese Bun (small)	235

Shoney's

	Calories
Blue Plate Specials	
Cajun Whitefish	480
Sides/Condiments	
Mashed Potatoes/Gravy	220
Corn	175
Green Beans	125
Cranberry Sauce, 1.5 oz	65
Breakfast Menu Selections	
All Star Breakfast (add options)	190
Breakfast Sides	
Bacon (3 strips)	120
Grits - 4 oz	105
White Toast – 2 slices w/maragine	200
Wheat Toast – 2 slices w/margarine	190
Sourdough Toast – 2 slices w/margarine	205
Apple Cinnamon Jelly – 1 packet	35
Grape Jelly – 1 packet	35
Strawberry Jam – 1 packet	35
Margarine - 1 packet (5 g)	35
Creamer, Half & Half® – 1 Container (15 g)	20
Add-Ons/Sides	
Bacon – per slice	40
BBQ Sauce – per 1.5 oz	70
Cocktail Sauce – per 1.5 oz	55
Grilled Onions – 1.5 oz	70

Sauteed Mushrooms – 3 oz	105
Secret Sauce – per 1.5 oz	170
Sweet & Sour Sauce – per 1.5 oz	70
Swiss Cheese – 1 slice	160

Junior Meals

Junior Chicken	190
Junior Fish & Chips	310

Salad

Dave's Pasta – 2/3 Cup	170
Potato, Classic – 1/2 Cup	190

Seafood

Grilled Cod, Lite	200
Grilled Salmon, Lite	180
Grilled Shrimp, Lite	320

Seafood Bar

Cheese, Deli Shred – 1 Tblsp	70
Cheese, Parmesan – 1 Tblsp	20
Cole Slaw – 1/4 Cup	125
Corn, Seasoned – 4 oz	175
Crackers, Club – 1 Packet (7 g)	30
Crackers, Oyster – 10 Crackers	180
Crackers, Saltines – 1 Packet (5.9 g)	25
Gravy, Brown – 2 oz	35
Margarine – Individual	35
Pinto Beans – 4 oz	135
Rolls, Yeast – each	115

Skyline Chili

Item	Calories
Black Beans And Rice	330
Cheese Coney	350
Chili Plain (regular)	250
Chili Plain w/Beans (regular)	260
Chili Sandwich	190
Chili Sandwich w/cheese	300
Coney (regular)	240
Garden Salad (large)	150
Garden Salad (regular)	80
Greek Salad (regular)	370
Kid-Sized SkyFries	210

SouperSalad

Dressing	Calories
Blue Cheese	130
Fat-Free Cranberry Vinaigrette	10
Fat-Free French Dressing	30
Fat-Free Italian w/Cheese	15
French Dijon Mustard	10
Gourmet Mayonnaise	100

SOUPERSALAD – STEAK ESCAPE

Greek Dressing	100
Green Goddess	130
Honey Mustard	120
Hot Bacon	140
House Vinaigrette	110
Tableside Caesar	140
Tangy Oriental	70
Thousand Island	150

Soup

Beef Stroganoff	350
Chicken Creole	320
Chicken Tetrazini	350
Cream of Cauliflower	190
Cream of Mushroom	225
Cream of Spinach	80
German Potato	320
Hungarian Mushroom	350
Mac and Cheese	350
Mama Mia Chicken	320
New England Clam Chowder	290
Potato Leek	255
Santa Fe Chicken	320
Shrimp Creole	255
Tomato Basil	225
Mexican Corn Chowder	225
Mushroom Cheese Soup	255
Potato Corn Chowder	320

Bread

Cornbread	60
Garlic Bread Stick	120
Jalapeno Cheddar Focaccia	70
Mediterranean Focaccia	70

Steak Escape

7" Sandwiches	Calories
Hambrosia	490
Vegetarian	500

Kids Sandwiches

Steak & Cheese	260
Chicken & Cheese	255
Turkey & Cheese	235
Ham & Cheese	235
All White-Meat Tenders (2)	240

Salads

Side Salad	190
Grilled Salad w/steak	340
Grilled Salad w/chicken	330
Grilled Salad w/turkey	285
Grilled Salad w/ham	285

LOWER CALORIES

STEAK ESCAPE – SUBWAY

Toppings

Provolone Cheese	105
Swiss Cheese	100
Cheddar Cheese	115
American Cheese – white	100
Mayonnaise	100
Brown Mustard	0
BBQ Sauce	40
Italian Dressing	50
Ranch Dressing	85
Margarine	205
Sour Cream	60
Lettuce	0
Tomato	25
Mild Peppers	10
Jalapeno Peppers	10
Black Olives	30
Bacon	80

Subway

Sandwiches	Calories
6" Ham	290
6" Roast Beef	290
6" Roasted Chicken Breast	320
6" Steak & Cheese	390
6" Subway Club®	320
6" Turkey Breast	280
6" Turkey Breast & Ham	290
6" Veggie Delite®	230
Double Meat Ham	350
Double Meat Roast Beef	360
Double Meat Turkey Breast	340
Double Meat Turkey Breast & Ham	360
Gardenburger®	390
Ham on Deli Round	210
Honey Mustard Ham	310
Lloyd's BBQ Chicken	330
Red Wine Vinaigrette Club	350
Roast Beef on Deli Round	220
Sweet Onion Chicken Teriyaki	380
Thai Sesame Chicken	370
Tuna on Deli Round	330
Turkey Breast on Deli Round	220
Veggi-Max	390

Salads	
Cold Cut Trio™	230
Ham	110
Italian BMT®	280
Meatball	330
Roast Beef	120

SUBWAY

Roasted Chicken Breast	140
Seafood & Crab®	200
Steak & Cheese	180
Subway Club®	150
Subway Melt®	200
Tuna	240
Turkey Breast	100
Turkey Breast & Ham	120
Veggie Delite®	50

Breakfast Sandwich On Deli Round

Bacon & Egg	320
Cheese & Egg	320
Ham & Egg	310
Steak & Egg	330
Vegetable & Egg	290
Western & Egg	300

Breakfast Sandwich On 6″ Italian Or Wheat Bread

Bacon & Egg	450
Cheese & Egg	440
Ham & Egg	430
Steak & Egg	460
Vegetable & Egg	410
Western & Egg	430

Omelets & French Toast

Bacon & Egg (1)	240
Cheese & Egg	240
French Toast w/syrup	350
Ham & Egg	230
Steak & Egg	250
Vegetable & Egg	210
Western & Egg	220

Soups (1 cup)

Black Bean	180
Brown and Wild Rice w/chicken	190
Cheese w/ham and bacon	230
Chicken and Dumpling	130
Chili Con Carne	310
Cream of Broccoli	130
Cream of Potato w/bacon	210
Minestrone	70
New England Style Clam Chowder	140
Potato Cheese Chowder	210
Roasted Chicken Noodle	90
Tomato Bisque	90
Vegetable Beef	90

Breads

6″ Hearty Italian	210
6″ Honey Oat	250
6″ Italian (White)	200
6″ Italian Herbs & Cheese	240

6" Monterey Cheddar	240
6" Parmesan Oregano	210
6" Roasted Garlic	230
6" Sourdough	210
6" Wheat	200
Deli Style Roll	170
Wrap	200

Sauces & Condiments

Bacon – 2 strips	45
Chipotle Southwest	90
Dijon Horseradish	90
Fat-Free French	70
Fat-Free Honey Mustard	30
Fat-Free Italian	20
Fat-Free Ranch	60
Fat-Free Red Wine Vinaigrette	30
Fat-Free Sweet Onion	40

Meats (amount on 6" Sub)

Cold Cut Trio™ Meats	140
Ham	60
Italian BMT® Meats	180
Meatball	240
Roast Beef	70
Roasted Chicken	90
Steak (no cheese)	90
Subway Club® Meats	100
Subway Seafood & Crab®	110
Tuna	150
Turkey Breast	50

Sweet Tomatoes & Souplantation

Salads (1 Cup)	Calories
Bartlett Pear & Walnut Salad	180
BBQ Julienne Chopped Salad	190
Caesar Salad Asiago	190
California Cobb Salad	180
Cape Cod Spinach w/walnuts	170
Chicken Tortilla Salad	180
Classic Antipasto Salad w/peppered salami	140
Ensalada Azteca Salad	130
Greek Salad	120
Italian Sub Salad w/turkey & salami	260
Mandarin Spinach Salad w/caramelized walnuts	170
Mediterranean Salad	150
Monterey Blue Salad w/peanuts	200
Pesto Orzo Salad w/pinenuts	220
Ragin' Cajun Salad	200
Ranch House BLT Salad w/turkey	180
Roasted Vegetables Salad w/feta & olives	140
Roma Tomato, Mozzarella & Basil Salad	120

SWEET TOMATOES & SOUPLANTATION

Smoked Turkey & Spinach Salad w/almonds	190
Sonoma Spinach Salad w/Honey Dijon Vinaigrette	210
Spiced Pecan & Roasted Vegetable	180
Spinach Gorgonzola w/spiced pecans	210
Strawberry Fields w/carmelized walnuts	130
Summer Lemon w/spiced pecans	220
Traditional Spinach Salad w/bacon	160
Watercress & Orange Salad	90
Won Ton Chicken Happiness	150

Dressings (2 Tblsp)

Bacon	120
Balsamic Vinaigrette	180
Basil Vinaigrette	160
Blue Cheese	140
Creamy Italian	120
Cucumber (reduced-calorie)	80
Fat Free Honey Mustard (fat-free)	45
Fat Free Italian (fat-free)	20
Fat Free Ranch (fat-free)	50
Garlic Parmesan Seasoned Croutons (low-fat, 5 pieces)	40
Honey Mustard	150
Kahlena French	120
Parmesan Pepper Cream	160
Ranch	130
Roasted Garlic	140
Thousand Island	110
Tomato Basil Croutons (5 Pieces)	45

Soup (1 Cup)

Albino Bean Chicken Cuisine	190
Albondigas Buenas (a meatball soup)	190
Arizona Chili	220
Be Wild With Mushroom	220
Big Chunk Chicken Noodle (low-fat)	160
Broc On	220
Butternut Squash Soup (vegetarian)	140
Chicken Fajitas & Black Bean Soup	280
Chicken Tortilla Soup w/Jalapeno Chiles & Tomatoes (Low Fat)	100
Chunky Potato Cheese Soup w/thyme	210
Country Corn & Red Potato Chowder	160
Cream of Broccoli Soup (vegetarian)	210
Cream of Chicken Soup	250
Cream of Mushroom Soup (non-vegetarian)	290
Creamy Vegetable Chowder	200
Deep Kettle House Chili (low-fat)	230
Deep Kettle House Chili w/ 33% more meat!	250
Devotion to The Ocean	220
Do The Stew!	280
Do The Stew! w/barley	290
El Paso Lime & Chicken Soup	160

SWEET TOMATOES & SOUPLANTATION

French Onion Soup (low-fat)	80
Garden Fresh Vegetable Soup (low-fat)	110
Garlic Kickin Roasted Chicken	140
Green Chile Stew	150
Hungarian Vegetable (low-fat)	120
Irish Potato Leek Soup (vegetarian)	260
Living on the Veg	90
Lonely for Minestrone	150
Longhorn Beef Chili	190
Make Room for Mushroom	240
Manhattan Clam Chowder	130
Marvelous Minestrone Soup	210
Minestrone w/Italian sausage	210
Mulligatawny Soup	210
Navy Bean Soup w/Ham	340
Neighbor Joe's Gumbo	280
New Orleans Jambalaya	210
Not Skimpy on the Shrimpy	290
Old Fashion Vegetable Soup (low-fat/vegetarian/ no cholesterol)	100
Posole Soup	150
Potato Sprung a Leek	190
Rock N' Mole Chili	240
Santa Fe Black Bean Chili (low-fat/vegetarian)	190
Shrimp Bisque	300
Southwest Tomato Cream Soup	120
Spicy 4-Bean Minestrone (low-fat/vegetarian)	140
Spicy Sausage & Pasta Soup	310
Sweet Tomato Cream Soup	180
Sweet Tomato Onion Soup (low-fat/vegetarian)	110
Texas Red Chili	240
Three-Bean Turkey Chili (low-fat/high-fiber/non-dairy)	140
Tomato Parmesan & Vegetables (low-fat/vegetarian /dairy)	120
Toot Your Horn for Crab & Corn	290
Tortellini Soup	180
Turkey Vegetable Soup	270
Tuscany Chicken Stew	190
Vegetable Beef Stew	250
Vegetable Medley Soup (low-fat/vegetarian)	90
Vegetarian Chili (vegetarian)	150
Vegetarian Harvest Soup (vegetarian)	190
Vegetarian Lentils & Brown Rice (low-fat/vegetarian)	130
Veggie Jackson	100
Very Nice Chicken & Rice	160
Muffins & Breads (1)	
Apple Cinnamon Bran Muffin (96% Fat Free)	80
Apple Raisin Muffin	150
Banana Nut Muffin	150
Big Hearth Pizza Focaccia	140

SWEET TOMATOES & SOUPLANTATION – TCBY

Bruschetta Focaccia	130
Buttermilk Cornbread (low-fat)	140
Cappuccino Chip Muffin	160
Caribbean Key Lime Muffin	170
Carrot Pineapple Muffin w/oat bran	150
Cherry Nut Muffin	150
Chile Corn Muffin (Low Fat)	140
Chocolate Brownie Muffin	170
Chocolate Chip Muffin	170
Country Blackberry Muffin	170
Cranberry Orange Bran Muffin (96% fat-free)	80
Fruit Medley Bran Muffin (96% fat-ree)	80
Garlic Parmesan Focaccia (low-fat)	100
Georgia Peach Poppyseed Muffin	150
Indian Grain Bread (low-fat)	200
Lemon Muffin	140
Nutty Peanut Butter Muffin	170
Pauline's Apple Walnut Cake	180
Pepperoni Focaccia	180
Pumpkin Raisin Muffin	150
Roasted Potato Focaccia	150
Sauteed Vegetable Focaccia	150
Sourdough Bread (low-fat)	150
Strawberry Buttermilk Muffin	140
Sweet Orange & Cranberry Muffin	200
Taffy Apple Muffin	160
Tomatillo Focaccia	140
Tropical Papaya Coconut Muffin	180
Zucchini Nut Muffin	150

Pastas (1 Cup)

Bruschetta	260
Carbonara Pasta	280
Creamy Pepper Jack	290
Garden Vegetable w/meatballs	270
Greek Mediterranean	290
Italian Sausage w/red pepper puree	250
Italian Vegetable Beef	270
Lemon Cream & Asparagus	230
Macaroni & Cheese	260
Oriental Green Bean & Noodle (low-fat)	240
Tuscany Sausage w/capers & olives	240
Vegetable Ragu	250
Vegetarian Marinara w/basil	260

TCBY

Soft Serve Frozen Yogurt (1/2 Cup)	**Calories**
Non-fat	110
No Sugar Added, Non-fat	90
96% Fat Free	140
Non-fat & Non-dairy Sorbet	100

Taco Bell

Taco	Calories
Taco	170
Taco Supreme®	220
Soft Taco – Beef	210
Soft Taco – Chicken	190
Soft Taco Supreme® – Beef	260
Soft Taco Supreme® – Chicken	230
Grilled Steak Soft Taco	280
Double Decker® Taco Supreme®	280
Gordita	
Gordita Supreme® – Beef	310
Gordita Supreme® – Chicken	290
Gordita Supreme® – Steak	290
Gordita Baja® – Beef	350
Gordita Baja® – Chicken	320
Gordita Baja® – Steak	320
Gordita Nacho Cheese – Beef	300
Gordita Nacho Cheese – Chicken	270
Gordita Nacho Cheese – Steak	270
Chalupa	
Chalupa Supreme – Beef	390
Chalupa Supreme – Chicken	370
Chalupa Supreme – Steak	370
Chalupa Nacho Cheese – Beef	380
Chalupa Nacho Cheese – Chicken	350
Chalupa Nacho Cheese – Steak	350
Burritos	
Bean	370
Chili Cheese	390
Fiesta Burrito – Beef	390
Fiesta Burrito – Chicken	370
Fiesta Burrito – Steak	370
Specialties	
Tostada	250
Enchirito® – Beef	380
Enchirito® – Chicken	350
Enchirito® – Steak	360
MexiMelt®	290
Breakfast	
Breakfast Gordita	380
Breakfast Quesadilla	400
Breakfast Steak Quesadilla w/Green Sauce	460

Taco John's

Tacos	Calories
Chicken Softshell Taco	200
Crispy Taco	190

TACO JOHN'S – TACO TIME

Sierra Taco™ - Chicken	470
Softshell Taco	230
Taco Bravo®	360
Taco Burger	280
Burritos	
Bean Burrito	380
Beefy Burrito	440
Chicken & Potato Burrito	470
Combination Burrito	410
Super Burrito	450
Specialties	
Cheese Quesadilla	480
Chicken Festiva Salad w/o dressing	390
Sides	
Mexican Rice	250
Side Salad	290
Texas-Style Chili	280
Local Favorites	
Bean Tostada	160
Cheese Crisp	220
Chicken Fajita Burrito	350
Chilito	440
El Grande Chicken Taco	360
El Grande Taco	480
Mexi Rolls®	460
Ranch Burrito - Beef	440
Ranch Burrito - Chicken	410
Sierra Chicken Sandwich	480
Tostada	200

Taco Time

	Calories
Burritos	
Chicken & Black Bean	400
Crisp Bean	430
Crisp Chicken	420
Soft Bean	380
Soft Meat	490
Veggie	490
Tacos	
1/2 lb. Chicken Soft Taco	385
Crisp Taco	295
Soft Taco	315
Salads	
Chicken Fiesta	390
Chicken Taco	370
Nachos	
Cheddar Melt	205
Sides	
Mexi-Rice	160

LOWER CALORIES

TACO TIME – TIM HORTON

Sauces
Thousand Island Dressing	120
Green	5
Original Hot	10
Salsa Fresca	65

Tim Horton

Muffins	Calories
Blueberry Bran	300
Chocolate Chip	390
Low-fat Carrot	260
Low-fat Cranberry	260
Low-fat Honey	290
Oatbran Carrot 'n' Raisin	340
Oatbran 'n' Apple	350
Raisin Bran	360
Wild Blueberry	330

Bagels	
Blueberry	300
Cinnamon Raisin	300
Everything	300
Multigrain	300
Onion	295
Plain	290
Poppy Seed	300
Sesame Seed	300
Whole Wheat & Honey	300

Baked Goods	
Cheese Croissant	240
Croissant	210
Raisin Tea Biscuit	250
Tea Biscuit	220

Cream Cheese	
Garden Vegetable	150
Light	90
Plain	140
Strawberry	150

Beverages	
English Toffee Cappuccino	130
French Vanilla Cappuccino	130
Hot Chocolate	200

Sandwiches	
Albacore Tuna Salad	350
Chunky Chicken Salad	380
Fireside Roast Beef	470
Garden Vegetable	460
Harvest Turkey Breast	470

Soup (10 oz)	
Chicken Noodle	100

TIM HORTON – WENDY'S

Cream of Broccoli	190
Hearty Vegetable	130
Minestrone	125
Potato Bacon	195
Turkey & Wild Rice	120
Vegetable Beef Barley	110

Togo's

Sandwiches (Regular)	Calories
Albacore Tuna	450
Salads	
Farmer's Market	110
Oriental Chicken	370
Roasted Chicken Caesar	320
Soup (Large)	
Black Bean	270
Broccoli Cheese	270
Chicken Noodle	240
Chili	200
New England Clam Chowder	200
Turkey Pot Pie Soup	270
Dressing (1 Pouch) & Sides	
Low-fat Balsamic Vinegrette	100
Ranch	200
Potato Salad (single)	170

Wendy's

Sandwiches	Calories
Classic Single® w/everything	410
Jr. Hamburger	270
Jr. Cheeseburger	310
Jr. Bacon Cheeseburger	380
Jr. Cheeseburger Deluxe	350
Hamburger, Kids' Meal	270
Cheeseburger, Kids' Meal	310
Grilled Chicken Sandwich	300
Chicken Breast Fillet Sandwich	430
Spicy Chicken Sandwich	430
Salads	
Caesar Side Salad	70
Homestyle Garlic Croutons –1 packet	70
Caesar Dressing – 1 packet	150
Side Salad	35
Chicken BLT Salad	310
Homestyle Garlic Croutons – 1 packet	70
Honey Mustard Dressing – 1 packet	280
Mandarin Chicken™ Salad	150
Roasted Almonds – 1 packet	130
Crispy Rice Noodles – 1 packet	60

LOWER CALORIES

Oriental Sesame Dressing – 1 packet	250
Spring Mix Salad	180
Honey Roasted Pecans – 1 packet	130
House Vinaigrette Dressing – 1 packet	190
Taco Supremo Salad	360
Taco Chips – 1 packet	220
Sour Cream – 1 packet	60
Salsa – 1 each	30
Dressings (1 Packet)	
Fat-free French Style	80
Low-fat Honey Mustard	110
Reduced-fat Creamy Ranch	100
Stuffed Baked Potatoes	
Plain	310
Sour Cream & Chives	370
Whipped Margarine – 1 packet	60
Chili	
Small	200
Large	300
Cheddar Cheese – 1 packet, shredded (2 Tblsp)	70
Saltine Crackers – 2 each	25
Hot Chili Seasoning – 1 packet	5
Crispy Chicken Nuggets	
5 Piece	220
4 Piece Kids' Meal	180
Barbecue Sauce – 1 packet	40
Honey Mustard Sauc – 1 packet	130
Sweet & Sour Sauce – 1 packet	45
Frosty	
Junior	170

Whataburger

Sandwiches	Calories
Grilled Chicken	475
Justaburger	310
Kids Justaburger	305
Whataburger Jr	315
Whatacatch	470
Other Items	
Chicken Strips – 2 Pieces	380
Grilled Chicken Fajita Taco	365
Kids Chicken Strips	380
Salads	
Chicken Strips	420
Garden	50
Garden w/Cheddar cheese	215
Garden w/cheese & bacon	290
Grilled Chicken	230
Grilled Chicken w/Cheddar cheese	400
Seasoned Croutons – 1 packet	35

WHATABURGER – WHITE CASTLE

Dressings – 1 packet

Low-fat Ranch	65
Low-fat Vinaigrette	35
Salad Dressing (Large sandwich)	55
Salad Dressing (Small sandwich)	30

Sides

American Cheese Slice (large sandwich)	90
American Cheese Slice (small sandwich)	45
Bacon (breakfast & small sandwich)	75

Breakfast

Biscuit w/bacon	375
Biscuit	300
Breakfast on a Bun w/bacon	400
Breakfast on a Bun Ranchero w/bacon	405
Breakfast on a Bun Ranchero w/sausage	545
Egg Sandwich	320
Grape Jelly	35
Hashbrown Sticks	140
Honey – 1 packet	25
Margarine – 1 packet	25
Pancake Syrup – 1 packet	120
Strawberry Jam – 1 packet	40
Taquito w/bacon & egg	390
Taquito w/bacon, egg & cheese	430
Taquito w/potato & egg	380
Taquito w/potato, egg & cheese	430
Taquito w/sausage & egg	390
Taquito w/sausage, egg & cheese	435
Texas Toast	330

White Castle

Item	Calories
Hamburger	140
Cheeseburger	160
Double Hamburger	240
Double Cheeseburger	290
Bacon Cheeseburger	200
Fish Sandwich	180
Chicken Sandwich	200
Breakfast Sandwich	340
Chicken Rings	215
French Fries – small	115
Shake, Vanilla	350
Shake, Chocolate	330

LOWER CALORIES

192

VISIT DR. SMITH ONLINE

Thank you for losing weight with Dr. Smith. For more valuable information about the Dr. Smith Get Thin Program™ and weight loss products, visit our Web site at *www.DrSmithProgram.com* — no matter if you have just started losing weight or are looking to maintain what you have lost.

When visiting, you can:

- Sign up for e-mail special offers
- Shop online for Dr. Smith products — safely and securely
- Take advantage of one of our popular combination packages
- Learn more about the Dr. Smith Get Thin Program™

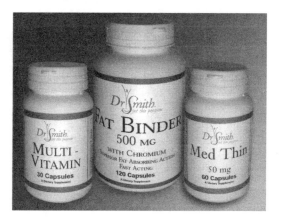

ALSO FROM DR. SMITH...

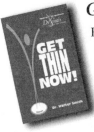

Get Thin Now!

For the first time, Dr. Smith reveals his time-tested Get Thin Program™ in this book! In *Get Thin Now!*, you will learn:

- How to enjoy a delicious variety of foods and still lose weight

- Eat 3 to 5 meals per day while losing

- Exercise is not essential for weight loss

- How to protect your new image as the weight comes off

And that's just the start! See for yourself why thousands of people are using Dr. Smith's Get Thin Program to lose the weight they want — and keep it off! Go online at *www.DrSmithProgram.com* to learn more.

Dr. Smith's Daily Diary

A perfect portable partner for tracking your monthly weight loss success.

- Stay in control of what you eat

- Easily record daily entries for all meals — including snacks

- Avoid worrying about daily weight entries

ALSO FROM DR. SMITH...

Perfect Companions

Dr. Smith provides safe, ephedra-free products that are designed to work hand-in-hand with your weight loss program.

Dr. Smith's Med Thin™
- Feel satisfied with less food*
- Maintain your lost weight*

Dr. Smith's Fat Binder™
- Protect yourself against* greasy, oily foods
- Use as a great companion when dining out

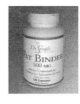

Dr. Smith's Multi-Vitamin
- Replenish essential nutrients during weight loss*
- Maintain your energy while losing weight*

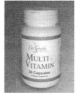

These products are available individually or in one of our popular packages. To order, simply go online at *www.DrSmithProgram.com*, or call toll-free 1-888-DOC-SMITH (1-888-362-7648).

*This statement has not been evaluated by the FDA. This product is not intended to diagnose, treat, cure or prevent any disease.

MY FAVORITE FOODS

Item   **Calories**

_____

_____

_____

_____

_____

_____

_____

_____

_____

_____

196 _____

_____

_____

_____

_____

_____

_____

_____

_____

_____

_____

_____

_____

MY FAVORITE FOODS

Item   Calories

_____

_____

_____

_____

_____

_____

_____

_____

_____

_____

_____

_____ **197**

_____

_____

_____

_____

_____

_____

_____

_____

_____

_____

_____

MY FAVORITE FOODS

Item   **Calories**

_____

_____

_____

_____

_____

_____

_____

_____

_____

_____

198 _____

_____

_____

_____

_____

_____

_____

_____

_____

_____

_____

MY FAVORITE FOODS

Item   **Calories**

_____

_____

_____

_____

_____

_____

_____

_____

_____

_____

_____

_____ **199**

_____

_____

_____

_____

_____

_____

_____

_____

_____

_____

_____

MY FAVORITE FOODS

Item   Calories

_____

_____

_____

_____

_____

_____

_____

_____

_____

_____

_____

200 _____

_____

_____

_____

_____

_____

_____

_____

_____

_____

_____

_____

MY FAVORITE FOODS

Item   Calories

--- **201**

MY FAVORITE FOODS

Item   **Calories**

_____

_____

_____

_____

_____

_____

_____

_____

_____

_____

202 _____

_____

_____

_____

_____

_____

_____

_____

_____

_____

_____

_____

MY FAVORITE FOODS

Item   **Calories**

_____

_____

_____

_____

_____

_____

_____

_____

_____

_____

_____

_____ **203**

_____

_____

_____

_____

_____

_____

_____

_____

_____

_____

_____

MY FAVORITE FOODS

Item   Calories

_____
_____
_____
_____
_____
_____
_____
_____
_____
_____
_____

204 _____
_____
_____
_____
_____
_____
_____
_____
_____
_____
_____
_____

MY FAVORITE FOODS

Item   **Calories**

_____

_____

_____

_____

_____

_____

_____

_____

_____

_____

_____ **205**

_____

_____

_____

_____

_____

_____

_____

_____

_____

_____

MY FAVORITE FOODS

Item   **Calories**

206
_____
_____
_____
_____
_____
_____
_____
_____
_____
_____
_____
_____
_____
_____
_____
_____
_____
_____
_____
_____
_____
_____
_____

MY FAVORITE FOODS

Item   Calories

_____

_____

_____

_____

_____

_____

_____

_____

_____

_____

_____ **207**

_____

_____

_____

_____

_____

_____

_____

_____

_____

_____

MY FAVORITE FOODS

Item   **Calories**

_____

_____

_____

_____

_____

_____

_____

_____

_____

_____

208 _____

_____

_____

_____

_____

_____

_____

_____

_____

_____

_____